The School Practitioner's Concise Companion
to Health and Well-Being

The School Practitioner's Concise Companion to Health and Well-Being

Edited by

Cynthia Franklin
Mary Beth Harris
Paula Allen-Meares

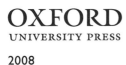

OXFORD
UNIVERSITY PRESS

2008

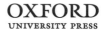

OXFORD
UNIVERSITY PRESS

Oxford University Press, Inc., publishes works that further
Oxford University's objective of excellence
in research, scholarship, and education.

Oxford New York
Auckland Cape Town Dar es Salaam Hong Kong Karachi
Kuala Lumpur Madrid Melbourne Mexico City Nairobi
New Delhi Shanghai Taipei Toronto

With offices in
Argentina Austria Brazil Chile Czech Republic France Greece
Guatemala Hungary Italy Japan Poland Portugal Singapore
South Korea Switzerland Thailand Turkey Ukraine Vietnam

Copyright © 2008 by Oxford University Press, Inc.

Published by Oxford University Press, Inc.
198 Madison Avenue, New York, New York 10016

www.oup.com

Oxford is a registered trademark of Oxford University Press

Library of Congress Cataloging-in-Publication Data

The school practitioner's concise companion to health and well-being / edited by
Cynthia Franklin, Mary Beth Harris, and Paula Allen-Meares.
p. cm.
Includes bibliographical references and index.
ISBN 978-0-19-537059-1
1. School hygiene. 2. School nursing. I. Franklin, Cynthia. II. Harris, Mary Beth.
III. Allen-Meares, Paula, 1948-
LB3405.S335 2009
371.7'12—dc22   2008018231

9 8 7 6 5 4 3 2 1
Printed in the United States of America
on acid-free paper

Preface

School-based practitioners are frequently called upon to address issues concerning the health and well-being of students. More than ever before we live in a society where health and mental health issues are recognized to intersect and risky behavioral practices during childhood are known to turn into serious health issues such as addictions, obesity, HIV infection, and even early death. No school practitioner is exempt from a need to have an armament of effective practices to prevent debilitating and self-destructive behaviors such as substance abuse, unsafe sexual practices, and eating disorders. Effective practices are especially needed to assist vulnerable and high-risk populations of students who may be predisposed to health-related problems through both their genetic history and social experiences. Practitioners are asking, what are the nuts and bolts of research-based information for addressing various health problems? *The School Practitioner's Concise Companion to Health and Well-Being* is a book designed to provide knowledge and practice-related information for timely issues that affect a student's health and well-being.

Contents of this Book

The School Practitioner's Concise Companion to Health and Well-Being was developed with the practicing school professional in mind. This companion book offers targeted content on how to improve the health of students through addressing high-risk behaviors. Contents of this book provide easy-to-read practice information, including case studies and practice guidelines to use when intervening with students, families, and school systems. A theme of several of the chapters in this companion book is prevention. Chapters in this book offer timely reviews of effective prevention programs and practices for important issues such as substance abuse, HIV infection, and sexually transmitted diseases. In addition, chapters cover important interventions for the potentially lethal conditions of self-harming and eating disorders that often plague today's youths. Finally, this companion book offers a chapter on how to design and use life skills groups, a practice approach that may be useful for a variety of behavioral and health-related problems. To add to the usefulness of the content of this book, each chapter follows a practice-friendly outline that includes the headings *Getting Started, What We Know, What We Can Do, Tools and Practice Examples, and Points to Remember,* thus providing a quick reference guide to information.

The *School Practitioner's Concise Companion to Health and Well-Being* is one of four companion books that were created to equip school professionals to effectively take action on social and health issues and mental health problems that are confronting schools. All four books in this series offer a quick and easy guide to information and solutions for today's pressing school problems. Content for the companion books was developed using chapters from Oxford's popular resource volume, *The School Services Sourcebook.* In contrast to the exhaustive and comprehensive *Sourcebook,* the briefer companion books are designed to provide succinct information for those who want to address a particular topic.

Objectives of the Companion Books

When planning the concise companion books, we had three main objectives in mind. Our first objective was to provide a series of affordable books whose content covered important and timely topics for school-based practitioners. We wanted the companion books to be like a search command on a computer where a quick search using a keyword or phrase can selectively lead you to the information you need. Each companion book contains updated knowledge tools and resources that can help practitioners quickly access information to address a specific problem area or concern. The second objective was for these books to communicate evidenced-based knowledge from research to practice but to do so in a way that practitioners could easily consume this knowledge. As editors, we wanted each chapter to be applied, providing practice examples and tools that can be used in day-to-day practice within a school.

A third objective was to create a series of practical books that school practitioners could use daily to guide their practices, prepare their presentations, and answer questions asked to them by teachers, parents, and administrators. For this reason, each chapter in these concise companion books on health and well-being is replete with quick reference tables, outlines, practice examples, and Internet resources for consultation.

How the Topics Were Selected

There are many important concerns facing today's schools and you may be wondering why we chose to address these particular health issues instead of a dozen other problem areas. School professionals who helped us create the timely topics addressed in this companion book provided selected topics. The original chapter topics in this book were identified through feedback from school social workers in six regions of the country. Social workers in California, Georgia, Michigan, New Mexico, Oregon, and Texas communicated with us through e-mail questionnaire, individual interviews, and focus groups. We asked about the overall challenges of working in a school setting. We asked about the most urgent and frequent problems school social workers and other practitioners encounter with students and families. School practitioners told us, for example, that their practice requires knowledge and skills for a variety of health-related, behavioral problems. A primary aspect of their work is direct services to individuals (school staff as well as students), to groups, and to families. Practitioners further told us that they need information on how to work with school professionals to interpret educational policies and design effective programs that will positively impact the health and well-being of students.

Acknowledgments

First and foremost we want to thank the Oxford University Press for supporting this work. Our deepest gratitude goes to Joan H. Bossert and Maura Roessner for their help and guidance in developing the companion books. In addition, we are thankful to Dr. Albert Roberts who gave us the inspiration and support to develop resource books for practitioners. We would further like to thank all from the team of professionals that worked on *The School Services Sourcebook*— Melissa Wiersema, Tricia Cody, Katy Shepard, and Wes Baker and our editorial board. Finally, we give credit to all the school social workers and school mental health professionals who participated in our survey and all those that informally gave us feedback on what topics to cover.

Cynthia Franklin, PhD
The University of Texas at Austin

Mary Beth Harris, PhD
Central Florida University

Paula Allen-Meares, PhD
The University of Michigan

Contents

Contributors

Tamara DeHay
Graduate Student
Department of Educational Psychology
University of Texas, Austin

Laura DiGiovanni
Graduate Student
School of Social Work
University of Texas, Austin

David R. Dupper, PhD
College of Social Work
University of Tennessee, Knoxville

Theresa J. Early, PhD
Associate Professor
College of Social Work
Ohio State University

Brooke Hersh
Graduate Research Assistant
College of Education
University of Texas, Austin

Lori K. Holleran, PhD
Assistant Professor
School of Social Work
University of Texas, Austin

Laura Hopson, MSSW
Graduate Research Assistant
School of Social Work
University of Texas, Austin

Soyon Jung
Graduate Student
School of Social Work
University of Texas, Austin

Reshma B. Naidoo, PhD
Graduate Student
Department of School Psychology
University of Texas, Austin

Matthew D. Selekman, MSW, LSW
Private Practice
Evanston, Illinois

Katherine Shepard
Graduate Student
Department of School Psychology
University of Texas, Austin

The School Practitioner's Concise Companion to Health and Well-Being

Substance Abuse Prevention

Effective School-Based Programs

Laura DiGiovanni

Getting Started

According to all of the latest figures, it appears that our youth are smoking cigarettes, drinking alcohol, and using illicit drugs *less* frequently (Substance Abuse and Mental Health Services Administration [SAMHSA], 2004). Children's attitudes have appeared to improve regarding substance use and abuse in recent years. In addition, participation in delinquent behaviors has dramatically declined in our youth. This is all good news and means that the substance abuse prevention approaches are working. However, many students in our schools continue to smoke cigarettes, drink alcohol under age, and use illicit drugs. If some children have changed, programs will need to be even more effective to reach the remaining potential users. Therefore, it is more important than ever that the programs we use are the most effective in school-based prevention programs. One program that appears to be effective is the Life Skills Training (LST) program.

The reality of substance use among our youth is still very striking. The National Institute on Alcohol Abuse and Alcoholism (NIAAA, 2004) identified alcohol as the primary psychoactive substance used by our youth. The Fiscal Year 2005 Congressional Budget Justification (NIAAA, 2004) indicates that 78% of 12th graders, 67% of 10th graders, and 47% of 8th graders have used alcohol. In addition, inhalant use among 8th graders shows a dramatic increase over the past year (SAMHSA, 2004). Although illicit drug use seems to have decreased in recent years, prescription drug use and abuse remains high (SAMHSA, 2004). Also, heroin and crack use by students has not declined and continue to present problems. According to the National Survey on Drug Use and Health (SAMHSA, 2004), 31% of children aged 12–17 years had smoked cigarettes in their lifetime. These statistics highlight the need for the use of *effective* substance abuse prevention approaches.

What We Know

Although prevention programs vary regarding focus (e.g., parents, family, and communities), substance abuse prevention programs have primarily been school based. Schools have the greatest access to the majority of the nation's children and are well known for providing education and collecting data from students about substance use and abuse (Burke, 2002).

Approaches to Substance Abuse Prevention

Traditional approaches to school-based substance abuse prevention have included information dissemination of facts, such as public service announcements. Fear arousal (e.g., trying to scare children into avoiding alcohol and drug use) is another commonly used method of traditional instruction. Another possible traditional approach has included moral appeals (e.g., doing the "right" thing). Finally, affective education, or focusing on children's feelings of self-worth and feelings about smoking, drinking, or using drugs, was included. However, none of these approaches has seemed to be successful. The main argument for the limited or complete lack of success suggests that these methods do not address the *underlying causes* of substance use and abuse (Botvin & Botvin, 1992; Gottfredson, 1996; Kinder, Pape, & Walfish, 1980; Schinke, Botvin, & Orlandi, 1991; Sherman, 2000; Swisher & Hoffman, 1975). One of the most well-known school-based substance abuse prevention programs is Project DARE (Drug Abuse Resistance Education), in which police officers go to schools and provide factual information to students. However, studies have indicated that it is not effective (Ennett, Tobler, Ringwalt, & Flewelling, 1994; Gottfredson, 1996; Rosenbaum & Hanson, 1998; Sherman, 2000).

Beginning in the 1970s, psychosocial approaches began to emerge, including resistance skills, psychological inoculation, and personal and social skills training. These approaches address more of the *causes* of substance abuse and have produced more promising results for reducing alcohol and marijuana use, increasing knowledge and impacts on attitudes, beliefs, and social-resistance skills (Best et al., 1984; Hops, Tildesley, & Lichtenstein, 1990; McAlister, Perry, Killen, Slinkard, & Maccoby, 1980; Schinke et al., 1991).

Meta-Analytic Reviews

Research suggests that these programs also have limitations. Early meta-analyses indicated that these previously employed school-based substance abuse prevention programs appeared to increase knowledge but did little to change attitudes and behaviors of students regarding drug use or abuse (Bangert-Drowns, 1988; Brunvold & Rundall, 1988; Tobler, 1986). Their findings also consistently point toward the need for an increased focus on psychosocial factors, such as school, family, media, and peer influences, and on personal competencies, cognitive expectancies, social skills, and psychological factors (Bangert-Drowns, 1988; Botvin & Botvin, 1992; Bruvold & Rundall, 1988; Tobler, 1986).

However, later analyses indicate that these meta-analytic reviews had a number of weaknesses. Bruvold (1993) indicates that these studies failed to meet a number of necessary criteria for current meta-analytic reviews: They were not comprehensive, did not use a systematic screening process to eliminate studies that were not equal or methodologically sound, did not use appropriate statistical techniques, and did not cover a specified time period.

More recent meta-analytic studies conducted in the 1990s used more sophisticated statistical analyses, more methodologically sound studies, and a more defined set of studies in the analysis (Bruvold, 1993; Tobler & Stratton, 1997; White & Pitts, 1998). These meta-analyses revealed that school-based prevention programs that addressed more psychosocial factors were more effective in changing attitudes and behaviors (Bruvold, 1993; Tobler & Stratton, 1997; White & Pitts, 1998). For example, Bruvold (1993) noted that programs that attempted to develop a student's ability to recognize social pressures to use drugs and ways to resist them, along with the ability to identify immediate social and physical consequences, were better able to change students' attitudes and behaviors. This was best accomplished through lengthier practice, role-playing, a public declaration not to use, and most important, through discussion, rather than through earlier lecture models. Tobler and Stratton (1997) also improved on previous meta-analyses and determined that the most effective school-based prevention programs were smaller in size (not held in auditoriums) and more interactive. They noted that failures in the programs could have been due to poor implementation. Finally, White and Pitts (1998) determined that prevention programs that increased their focus on social skills training improved students' abilities to change attitudes and behaviors, along with increasing their knowledge about drug use and misuse. Some of these social skills included a component of improving self-esteem, assertiveness and refusal skills, and life skills. In order for school-based prevention programs to be effective, an increased focus on the social aspects of students' lives and less of a traditional lecture approach seem to be the common elements that the more recent meta-analytic studies have in common (see Table 1.1).

What We Can Do

Many of these school-based substance abuse prevention programs continue today and can be accessed through the Internet. The Center for Substance Abuse Prevention (CSAP, 1999) has created a National Registry of Effective Prevention Programs (NREPP) to identify, review, and disseminate effective alcohol, tobacco, and other drugs (ATOD) prevention programs (see Table 1.2 for program access information).

Life Skills Training and Previous Research
In the late 1970s, an integrative approach to school-based substance abuse prevention was developed by Gilbert Botvin, called the Life Skills Training

Table 1.1 Descriptions of Meta-Analyses

Author: Tobler (1986)

Type of Prevention Intervention: A variety—mostly traditional, mostly affective educational, information dissemination

Substances Studies: 143 programs—a variety, including tobacco, alcohol, and marijuana

Populations: Adolescents—a variety, causing problems with findings. A variety of programs included in criteria (some students had drug problems, some had disciplinary problems, and some no problems at all)

Findings: Programs were most effective in increasing knowledge; minor improvements in reducing behaviors; even smaller effects in improving attitudes; found that peer programs were most effective in producing positive changes. Weak methodology

---

Author: Bangert-Drowns (1988)

Type of Prevention Intervention: Mostly traditional—affective educational programs, information dissemination

Substances Studies: Smoking prevention programs

Populations: Elementary school to college students—traditional students

Findings: Maintained support of previous findings—programs increase knowledge of substances. Changes in student attitudes were more statistically significant. Behaviors continued to show limited change. Peers in programs appear to impact changes more than didactic instruction

---

Author: Bruvold and Rundall (1988)

Type of Prevention Intervention: Mostly traditional—affective educational programs, information dissemination

Substances Studies: 19 programs—alcohol and tobacco

Populations: Adolescent school students

Findings: Increased knowledge, but failed to change attitudes or behaviors

---

Author: Bruvold (1993)

Type of Prevention Intervention: Psychosocial—personal and social skills training

Substances Studies: 94 programs—tobacco prevention, curricula mainly provided in schools

Populations: Adolescent school students

Findings: Behavioral effect sizes were found to be largest for interventions with a social reinforcement orientation, moderate for interventions with developmental or social norms orientation, and small for traditional orientation

(continued)

Table 1.1 *(Continued)*

Author: Tobler and Stratton (1997)

Type of Prevention Intervention: Psychosocial—personal and social skills training

Substances Studies: 120 programs—tobacco, alcohol, marijuana, and illicit drugs

Populations: 5th–12th graders

Findings: Most effective programs in changing adolescent drug use were interactive (groups C and D) and included comprehensive life skill training (CLST) or social influence training (SIT). Larger groups were less effective

Author: White and Pitts (1998)

Type of Prevention Intervention: Psychosocial—personal and social skills training

Substances Studies: 62 prevention programs

Populations: 71% school-based

Findings: Most effective programs were a mix of focused interventions (assertiveness skills, refusal skills, and normative education) and generic training (life skills, decision-making, problem-solving, goal-setting, and communication skills)

program (Botvin, Eng, & Williams, 1980). As a research program, this effective model has received extensive study for more than 20 years, with results indicating approximately a 50%–87% reduction in the prevalence of tobacco, alcohol, or illicit drug use (National Health Promotion Associates [NHPA], 2002). In a strategic plan, Botvin and colleagues have systematically studied the effectiveness of the LST program, using experimental and quasi-experimental, pre- and posttest designs. First, they focused on the program's effectiveness and produced a 75% reduction in the number of new student cigarette smokers (Botvin et al., 1980). Then, they examined the LST program with different providers (e.g., teachers, peer-led classes, and school staff) with continued success (Botvin & Eng, 1982; Botvin, Renick, & Baker, 1983).

Further studies examined and demonstrated the effectiveness of the LST program in targeting alcohol and other illicit drugs (Botvin, Baker, Dusenbury, Tortu, & Botvin, 1990; Botvin, Baker, Renick, Filazzola, & Botvin, 1984). When examining the effectiveness with different ethnicities (in particular, Hispanic and African American) and substances, findings not only supported the efficacy of the LST program but also determined that the program did not always require cultural modifications (Botvin et al., 1993; Botvin, Dusenbury, Baker, & James-Ortiz, 1989).

Botvin and his colleagues (1990) also examined the generalizability of the program by conducting a large-scale controlled prevention trial of 5,954 students in

Table 1.2 Overview of Major Preventive Approaches

Intervention	Focus	Methods	Source/Name of Education Program	Web Site
Traditional				
Information dissemination (fear arousal, moral appeals)	Increase knowledge of drugs, consequences of use; promote antidrug-use attitudes	Didactic instruction, discussion, audio/video presentations, displays of substances, posters, pamphlets, school assembly programs	Public-information campaigns; government agencies; community groups (e.g., American Cancer Society, National Council on Alcoholism)	American Cancer Society: http://www.cancer.org/docroot/PED/content/PED_I0_I4_How_to_Fight_Teen_Smoking.asp National Council on Alcoholism: http://www.ncadd-middlesex.com/
			Drug Abuse Resistance Education (DARE)	Drug Abuse Resistance Education: http://www.dare.com/home/default.asp
Affective education	Increase self-esteem, responsible decision making, interpersonal growth; generally includes little or no information about drugs	Didactic instruction, discussion, experiential activities, group problem-solving exercises	Here's Looking at You 2000 Me-Me	Here's Looking at You 2000: http://www.chef.org/prevention/looking.php Me-Me: http://www.ed.gov/pubs/EPTW/eptw9/eptw9m.html
Alternatives	Increase self-esteem, self-reliance; provide variable alternatives to drug use; reduce boredom and sense of alienation (arts, crafts, music, sports)	Organization of youth centers, recreational activities; participation in community services projects; vocational training	Outward Bound (wilderness program)	Outward Bound: http://www.outwardbound.org/

Psychosocial				
Resistance skills training	Increase awareness of social influence to smoke, drink, or use drugs; develop skills for resisting substance-use influences; increase knowledge of immediate negative consequences; establish non-substance-use norms	Class discussion; resistance skills training; behavioral rehearsal; extended practice via behavioral "homework"; use of same age or older peer leaders	Prevention Enhancement Protocols System (PEPS)	Prevention Enhancement Protocols System: http://www.health.org/govpubs/PHD822/aap.aspx
Personal and social skills training	Increase decision making, personal behavior change, anxiety reduction, communication, social and assertive skills; application of generic skills to resist substance-use influences	Class discussion; cognitive-behavioral skills training (instruction, demonstration, practice, feedback, reinforcement)	General personal and social skills (Caplan et al., 1992)	General Personal and Social Skills: http://www.ncbi.nlm.nih.gov/entrez/query.fcgi?cmd=Retrieve&db=PubMed&list_uids=1556286&dopt=Abstract
			Project Counseling Leadership About Smoking Pressure (CLASP)	Project CLASP: http://www.ssw.upenn.edu/crysp/publications/publ4_full.html
			Life Skills Training	Life Skills Training: http://www.lifeskillstraining.com/old3.cfm

Source: Adapted from Schinke et al. (1991, pp. 20–35).
Life Skills Training. Copyright © Gilbert J. Botvin, 1979–2004.

56 schools with positive results up to 40 months after the training. This research indicates the effectiveness of the LST program over a 6-year period with 7th, 8th, and 9th grade students (Botvin, Schinke, Epstein, Diaz, & Botvin, 1995). Given the number and variety of studies conducted on the LST program, it seems clear that it offers great opportunities for school-based substance abuse prevention.

Intervention With Steps and Examples

Based on a risk and protective model, the LST program has four main goals: to teach prevention-related information, to promote antidrug norms, to teach drug refusal skills, and to foster the development of personal self-management skills and general social skills (NHPA, 2002). The main objectives of the program are to

- provide students with the necessary skills to resist social (peer) pressures to smoke, drink, and use drugs;
- help them develop greater self-esteem, self-mastery, and self-confidence;
- enable children to effectively cope with social anxiety;
- increase their knowledge of the immediate consequences of substance abuse;
- enhance cognitive and behavioral competency to reduce and prevent a variety of health risk behaviors (NHPA, 2002).

Working solely with the students, the underlying assumption of the LST program is that substance abuse prevention needs to address a number of areas in a student's life. The program accomplishes this by addressing three major domains in its curriculum: drug resistance skills and information, self-management skills, and general social skills.

The drug resistance skills portion of LST provides information on the actual number of youth in the United States who use tobacco, alcohol, or illicit drugs, as well as the short- and long-term consequences of their usage (Botvin, 1996). Also included is "information about the declining social acceptability of cigarette smoking and other drug use, the physiological effects of cigarette smoking," how to avoid media pressures to smoke, drink, or use drugs; and how to resist peer pressure (Botvin, 1996, p. 223).

The personal self-management skills training encourages students to examine their self-image and how this impacts them, and how to problem solve while looking ahead at the consequences. Information on how to reduce stress, anxiety, and anger; how to identify problem situations, how to set goals; and how to self-monitor are also central to this domain (Botvin, 1996).

Finally, to empower students to overcome shyness, learn more effective communication skills, increase their assertiveness, and recognize their life choices, the LST program offers a general social skills component. This domain explores the topics of communication and socialization through both verbal and nonverbal skills. Through examining communication and socialization, issues about intimate relationships develop (Botvin, 1996).

The LST program spans 3 years of student development, typically either grades 6–8 or grades 7–9. The curriculum for the program has 15 sessions in the first year (7th grade), 10 sessions in the second year, and 5 sessions in the third year. Each session lasts approximately 45 minutes and can be taught either weekly or daily, depending on the students' needs. By reinforcing the information taught in the first year, the last 2 years are considered "booster" sessions in order to maintain the gains already established in the first year. The NHPA (2002) states that the entire curriculum must be taught in the sequence provided in order to gain the full benefits. The curriculum has been modified for elementary students (24 sessions, with 8 sessions per year), and studies continue with this population. Preliminary findings suggest that this curriculum modification is successful (Botvin et al., 2003) (see Table 1.3).

The standardized curriculum offers both teacher and student manuals, enabling providers (social workers, mental health professionals, teachers, school staff, and peers) to maintain the sequence of the curriculum and provide the instruction in a variety of settings. The teacher's manual includes goals, objectives, and lesson plans that detail the content and activities for each session. The student manuals have the necessary reference material, class exercises, and homework assignments for each session (Botvin, 1996).

Intervention methods used in the sessions include "didactic teaching methods, facilitation-group discussion, classroom demonstrations, and cognitive-behavioral skills training" (Botvin, 1996, p. 224). Because the majority of the sessions include facilitated group discussions, one of the main roles of the intervention provider is a skills trainer, or a coach, rather than an educator (Botvin, 1996).

The recommended ratio of students to provider is 25:1. In addition, studies have supported the curriculum being taught in a variety of settings, including school classrooms, after-school programs, summer camps, and community-based organizations (NHPA, 2002). However, NHPA indicates that a gymnasium is not an appropriate setting for students to learn the curriculum.

One of the strengths of the LST program is its simplicity, with easy-to-follow instructions for both teachers and students. Included in each LST program is a teacher's manual, student guide, and audiocassette tape with relaxation exercises (NHPA, 2002). The curriculum also offers evaluation tools, including pre- and post-tests, fidelity checklists (to monitor implementation by providers), and quizzes for the students. Teacher training in each curriculum level is highly recommended.

LST is a comprehensive coverage of a range of topics. The first year of the curriculum includes sessions on self-image and self-improvement; making

Table 1.3 Grid of Life Skills Program Structures for Elementary and Middle Schools

Program Levels	Elementary School Program Structure[a]	Program Levels	Middle School Program Structure[b]
Core curriculum: level 1	• 3rd or 4th grade • Composed of eight class sessions • Covers all skill areas	Core curriculum: level 1	• 6th or 7th grade • 15 class sessions • Cover all skill areas • Additional three class sessions on violence prevention (optional)
Core curriculum: level 2	• 4th or 5th grade • Eight class sessions • Reviews all skill areas	Booster session: level 2	• 7th or 8th grade • 10 class sessions • Additional two class sessions on violence prevention (optional)
Core curriculum: level 3	• 5th or 6th grade • Eight class sessions • Reviews all skill areas	Booster session: level 3	• 8th or 9th grade • Five class sessions • Additional two class sessions on violence prevention (optional)
Middle school general information	The booster sessions provide additional skill development and opportunities to practice in key areas. The beginning of each level depends upon the transition from elementary school to middle school/junior high school		
Elementary school general information	The elementary program can be used either alone or in combination with the middle school program. Under ideal conditions, it is intended to be implemented in a sequential manner across all 3 years of upper elementary school. However, the elementary program is designed to be flexible and can be implemented over 1, 2, or 3 years, depending on the availability of time		

Source: From the National Health Promotion Associates Web site: http://www.lifeskillstraining.com/program_structure1.cfm.
Life Skills Training. Copyright © Gilbert J. Botvin, 1979–2004.
[a] Entire program comprises 24 class sessions (approximately 30–45 minutes each) to be conducted over 3 years.
[b] Entire program comprises 30 class sessions (approximately 45 minutes each) to be conducted over 3 years.

decisions; the myths and realities of smoking, alcohol, and marijuana (the "gateway" drugs to more intense substance abuse); biofeedback and smoking; advertising; violence and the media; coping with anxiety and anger; communication skills; social skills; assertiveness training; and resolving conflicts. The second year exposes students to new topics, such as the causes and effects of drug abuse and violence, and resisting peer pressure. Topics expanded upon in this second year include making decisions, media influence, coping with anxiety and anger, communication skills, social skills, assertiveness training, and resolving conflicts. The final year builds on these basics, applying the knowledge to new situations that the students experience in which they have to cope.

Tools and Practice Examples

As indicated previously, each teacher's manual specifies the goals, objectives, materials needed, special preparation that may be required prior to the session, possible vocabulary that needs to be explained to the students, homework assignments to hand out, and then the actual directions on how to complete each session. A sample of the *Teacher Manual* material for the first social skills training session follows.

Social Skills (A)—Teacher Manual
Session Goal: To teach students basic social skills in order to develop successful interpersonal relationships.

Major Objectives
- Recognize that many people feel shy or uncomfortable in social situations.
- Discuss how shyness can be overcome.
- Practice making social contacts.
- Practice giving and receiving compliments.
- Practice initiating, sustaining, and ending conversations.

Materials Needed
- *Student Guide*
- Tennis balls (two or three)

Special Preparation
- None

Vocabulary
- Self-confident
- Specific

- Initiating
- Sustain
- Compliment

Homework

- *Student Guide*: Review *Getting Over Being Shy* (p. 71) and fill out *Social Activities Worksheet 21* (p. 76)

Introduction

Tell students that today you are going to cover some techniques that can help make them more socially attractive and self-confident. Many people are shy and uncomfortable in social situations, not because there is anything wrong with them, but simply because they have not learned the basic ingredients of social life.

Overcoming Shyness

1. Begin a discussion on shyness by asking students how many of them consider themselves to be shy or have been told that they were shy.
2. Ask students the following questions:
   (a) How many of you have been uncomfortable in social situations?
   (b) Why do people feel shy or uncomfortable in social situations?
   (c) Is there anything that you can do about it?
3. Tell students that many actors and well-known personalities are shy and uncomfortable being themselves but are comfortable and able to overcome their shyness by "acting" or playing a role. By learning social skills and practicing in situations that are fairly easy at first, they can develop social self-confidence. In the beginning, it helps to "act." They should develop "scripts" for various social situations and rehearse them (e.g., practice in front of a mirror).
4. Review strategies for getting over being shy (refer students to p. 71 of the *Student Guide*).

Getting Over Being Shy

Learn to act: You can learn new social skills and become more self-confident by handling difficult social situations as if you were a performer playing a role. For many shy people, it is easier to pretend they are someone else playing a part than it is to be themselves. Thus, thinking of yourself as an actor playing a part is a good *first step* in acquiring new social skills and becoming more confident. Start small and strive for gradual improvement: Begin by practicing on easy situations, gradually working up to more difficult ones. Develop scripts: Write out a brief script of what you want to say, how you want to say it, and what you want to do in each situation you are trying to master.

Practice: Rehearse at home. Practice the skills you are learning and how to handle specific situations using the scripts you developed. Watch yourself in the mirror and listen to your voice. If you can, practice with someone playing the part of the other person. Be persistent: Keep at it. If you stick to it and continue to work on improving, you are bound to succeed.

Points to Make

- Shyness can be overcome by learning to "act" as if you are not shy (by being more outgoing) and by improving your basic social skills.
- Anxiety about social contacts can be overcome by practicing the techniques learned in the *Coping with Anxiety* session, particularly mental rehearsal and deep breathing.

Initiating Social Contacts

1. Tell students that an important step in overcoming shyness and a valuable social skill involves initiating social contacts (saying hello or starting a conversation).
2. Calling someone they do not know very well on the phone and asking them for specific information. For example:
   (a) Call the operator to ask for phone numbers.
   (b) Call the local department store to ask about some product(s).
   (c) Call your friend and talk to his or her mom on the phone.
3. *Note:* It helps to have a telephone for these exercises.
4. Have students practice greeting people by saying hello or by nodding, waving, smiling, etc. Have students suggest other greetings and write them on the board. Have them rehearse some of these. For example, pairs of students can rehearse:
   (a) meeting in the hall
   (b) sitting down in the cafeteria
5. Have students practice asking directions from someone they do not know.
6. Practice starting conversations with new people in public places (e.g., movie and grocery lines, doctor's office, sporting events). Go over the examples in the *Student Guide* on *Meeting New People* p. 72 and have the students suggest additional "openers" from their own experience. Sample "openers":
   (a) "This line is so long, this must be a good movie."
   (b) "Have you heard anything about it?"
   (c) "Is that a good book? What's it about?"
   (d) "That's a nice jacket. Where did you get it?"
   (e) "Did you see the game last night? Who won?"

(Adapted from http://www.lifeskillstraining. com/pdf/Sample_Teachers_Manual.pdf)

Social Skills (A)—Student Manual

Accompanying the teacher's manual is a student manual that has information and material for each session. However, the student manuals contain more of the exercise materials, rather than the "nuts and bolts" of the items to be covered. A sample of the *Student Manual* material for the first social skills training session follows:

Getting Over Being Shy

Many people, even famous TV and movie personalities, can be shy and feel uncomfortable in social situations. However, you can learn to be more comfortable in social situations by learning how to deal with anxiety and nervousness (practiced in the last session) and by improving your social skills in social situations. Some ideas are listed here:

Learn to "act": You can learn new social skills and become more self-confident by "playing" a social situation as if you were an actor acting out a specific role.

Start small: Begin by practicing on easy situations, gradually working up to more difficult ones.

Prepare yourself: Write out a brief script and rehearse it at home, watch yourself in the mirror, and listen to your voice. This is what actors in plays and movies do.

Saying Hello

1. Another way to get over being shy is to practice saying hello to people.
2. Below are some common greetings:
   (a) "Hello" or "Hi"
   (b) "How is it going?"
   (c) "Good to see you."
   (d) "Have a good (nice) day."
3. Gestures (a nod, smile, or wave)
4. Get in the habit of saying hello to people. The more people you say hello to, the more people will say hello to you. Most people are shy. You can help them by saying hello first.

Meeting New People

Try to meet a lot of new people. Begin a conversation wherever you go (e.g., while standing in line at the movies, grocery store, bank, a sporting event, etc.). Start the conversation with something you have in common. Again, asking questions is an effective method. Below are some examples:

• "This line is so long, this must be a good movie. Have you heard anything about it?"
• "Is that a good book? What's it about?"

- "That's a nice jacket. Where did you get it?"
- "Did you see the game last night? Who won?"

(Life Skills Training. Copyright © Gilbert J. Botvin, 1979–2004.)

Resources

Resources for school-based substance abuse prevention programs can be found in the following list. The Web sites included in the list provide information regarding training manuals, video training tools, Web resources, books, journals, and journal articles.

Life Skills Training
National Health Promotion Associates, Inc.
711 Westchester Avenue
White Plains, NY 10604
(800) 293–4969
lstinfo@nhpanet.com

Life Skills Research
Institute for Prevention Research, Cornell University Medical College
411 East 69th Street, KB-201
New York, NY 10021
(212) 746–1270
ipr@mail.med.cornell.edu

Center for Substance Abuse Prevention
P.O. Box 2345
Rockville, MD 20847–2345
(800) 729–6686 or (240) 276–2130
http://www.prevention.samhsa.gov/

National Institute on Alcohol Abuse and Alcoholism
5635 Fishers Lane, MSC 9304
Bethesda, MD 20892–9304
http://www.niaaa.nih.gov/

National Institute on Drug Abuse
6001 Executive Boulevard, Room 5213
Bethesda, MD 20892–9561
(301) 443–1124
http://backtoschool.drugabuse.gov/

Substance Abuse and Mental Health Services Administration
P.O. Box 2345
Rockville, MD 20847–2345
(800) 729–6686 or TDD (hearing impaired): (800) 487–4889
http://www.samhsa.gov/ or www.health.org
e-mail: info@health.org

National Clearing House for Drug and Alcohol Information (NCADI)
11420 Rockville Pike
Rockville, MD 20852
(800) 729–6686
http://www.health.org

United States Department of Health and Human Services
200 Independence Avenue, S.W.
Washington, DC 20201
(877) 696–6775 or (202) 619–0257
http://www.os.dhhs.gov/

Provides Some Online Training
Drug and Alcohol Treatment and Prevention Global Network
http://www.drugnet.net/prevention.htm

Key Points to Remember

- Even though substance abuse has begun declining in recent years, tobacco, alcohol, and illicit drug use continues to plague our youth. Although a number of substance abuse prevention programs have been tried in the past, traditional models do not seem effective and have had poor outcomes. More recent models that include psychosocial components have had better outcomes and seem to be reducing substance use in children and adolescents.
- One of the most promising substance abuse prevention programs to date is the LST program. This program spans three grades for students, the first of which is intended to provide the foundation materials, and the last two of which are meant as "booster sessions" and are intended to maintain the progress made in the first year. Research has supported the effectiveness of this model, which continues to have positive study outcomes.
- One of the reasons for LST's effectiveness is its simplicity of use. Each session has been broken down for the teacher and student, enabling the structure of the program to be flexible for use with a number of different providers in a variety of settings. The simple, yet clear, manuals make it easy and effective to use.

Substance Abuse at Elementary Age

2

Effective Interventions

Soyon Jung
Lori K. Holleran

Getting Started

Substance use/abuse is usually perceived as a problem of the adult and adolescent population and seldom seriously examined with regard to elementary school children. According to Parents' Resource Institute for Drug Education (PRIDE, 2003), however, it is not uncommon among elementary school children to experiment with various substances. The PRIDE survey analyzing data collected from 72,025 students from 4th through 6th grade reported that 2.7% of 4th graders, 4.4% of 5th graders, and 5.6% of 6th graders smoked cigarettes during the previous year. The proportion of the elementary school students who drank beer or wine coolers in the previous year ranged from 6.3% (beer consumption among 4th graders) to 11.2% (wine coolers consumption among 6th graders). Substance use by elementary school children is not limited to tobacco or alcohol beverages. Three percent of 4th graders, 3.3% of 5th graders, and 3.9% of 6th graders reported inhalant use in the previous year. The percentage of the students using marijuana in the previous year ranged from 0.7% for 4th graders to 1.8% for 6th graders.

In addition to the prevalence of substance use/abuse among elementary school children, it should be noted that the age of first substance use is getting lesser (American Academy of Pediatrics, 1998). For example, the proportion of students who drank alcohol before the age of 13 years was about 16% for 11th- and 12th-grade males, but it was 33.3% for 10th-grade males (Centers for Disease Control and Prevention, 2004). It should be taken seriously because earlier onset of substance use is significantly related to heavier use and more addictive symptoms in later years, as well as more difficult rehabilitation if a problem emerges (Jenson & Howard, 1991; Knowles, 2001; Sarvela, Monge, Shannon, & Newrot, 1999). Early use of substances also has a physiological risk. A child's brain is different from an adult's and the deleterious effects of alcohol on a developing brain are profound (Kuhn, Swartzwelder, & Wilson, 1998).

These statistics and trends of experimentation with substances might suggest that substance use/abuse prevention programs be provided to elementary school students. There is also empirical evidence that well-designed prevention programs for elementary school children significantly reduce various problem behaviors, including substance use/abuse in their later lives (e.g., Hawkins, Catalano, Kosterman, Abbott, & Hill, 1999). Elementary school is often regarded as the ideal setting for substance use/abuse prevention programs (Gibson, Mitchell, & Basile, 1993). The reasons can be summarized as follows: First, the school environment has a powerful influence on children, given the time spent, learning process, and social interaction (St. Pierre, Mark, Kaltreider, & Campbell, 2001). Second, schools are the major provider of mental health services for children (Rones & Hoagwood, 2000), and a number of school-based prevention programs have been found effective (Gibson et al., 1993). Thus, many schools already have valuable resources and accumulated know-how regarding mental health services. Finally, students are more likely to obtain information about substances and talk about drugs with their schoolteachers rather than with their own parents (Alcoholism & Drug Abuse Weekly, 1999, April 19).

In this chapter, the authors present an overview of selective prevention interventions, a risk and protective factor paradigm, and two examples of evidence-based programs, the Strengthening Families Program (SFP) and Positive Action (PA). The two programs are particularly worth noting because they illustrate how preventive intervention can address risk, enhance protective factors, and be effectively implemented at school settings. Lastly, practical guidelines are presented for school social workers and other school mental health professionals who envision substance use/abuse prevention targeting elementary school children.

What We Know

Understanding Selective Prevention Programs

Preventive interventions are often classified into three categories, universal, selective, and indicated prevention, based on the target populations. Universal preventions address the entire population of a community or an organization such as an elementary school. Indicated preventions are directed toward specific individuals who are showing serious precursors or are already involved in problem behavior(s) such as substance use/abuse. On the other hand, selective prevention targets "subsets of the total population that are deemed to be at risk for substance abuse by virtue of their membership in a particular population segment—for example, children of adult alcoholics, dropouts, or students who are failing academically" (National Institute on Drug Abuse [NIDA], 1997b, p. 11). Selective prevention interventions are recommendable in elementary school settings, given that a majority of elementary school students do not exhibit substance use/abuse problem, but a significant number of them are exposed to multiple risk factors.

Program Goal and Theoretical Background of Selective Prevention

The ultimate goal of selective prevention is to deter the onset of substance abuse among at-risk groups and to help them be equipped with proper skills and information so that they can reduce their vulnerability (NIDA, 1997a). Based on a risk and protective factor model, selective prevention approaches usually pursue such goals by minimizing the impacts of risk factors and maximizing the effects of protective factors. Initially, risk factors for substance use/abuse were limited to a narrow range of factors such as biological or psychological variables only (Jenson, 1997). Recently, however, the risk factor model is usually grounded in comprehensive ecological frameworks. Table 2.1 shows some examples of

Table 2.1 Risk Factors from Multidimensional Perspectives	
	Study Number (see below for reference)
Individual	
Problematic health status (physical and mental)	2, 3, 4[a]
Constitutional factors/sensation-seeking orientation/ (genetic predisposition to chemical dependency)	1, 2, 3, 5[a]
Poor impulse control	3, 5[a]
Greater levels of rebelliousness	
Attention deficits	3
Early and persistent antisocial behavior/rebellious attitudes	1, 2, 5[a]
Early initiation of the problem behavior	1, 5[a]
Favorable attitudes toward the problem behavior	
Delinquency (e.g., history of trouble with the police)	
Decreased perception of risk	5[a]
Lack of social bonding/alienation	2, 5[a]
Family	
Family conflict/marital discord	1, 2, 3, 5[a]
Family stress	4[a]
Family disruption and/or dysfunction due to death, divorce, and parental incarceration	4[a]
Poor parent–child bonding	3
Poor parental supervision	5[a]
Poor family management practices/discipline	1, 2, 3, 5[a]
Family communication	3
Family history of mental health problem	4[a]

(continued)

Table 2.1 *(Continued)*

	Study Number (see below for reference)
Family present use or history of substance use/abuse	3, 4[a], 5[a]
Family history of problem behavior	1, 2
Favorable parental attitudes/parental permissiveness toward the problem behavior/substance use	1, 2, 5[a]
Incidence of child abuse, neglect, and trauma	2, 5[a]
Lack of support for positive school values and attitudes	4[a]
Economic deprivation	5[a]
Differential family acculturation	5[a]

Peers

Rejection by conforming peer group/alienation and Rebelliousness	1, 3
Association with drug-using peers/friends who engage in the problem behavior	1, 3, 5[a]
Alienation and rebelliousness	1, 2
Peer pressure	
Peer approval of drug use	

School

School failure/academic failure/beginning in late elementary school	1, 3, 5[a]
Low commitment to school	1, 2, 3
Absenteeism and dropout	2, 5[a]
Lack of cultural grounding and resources, language difficulties, or both	2
Dysfunction within the school environment such as high rates of substance abuse or unsafe school environment	4[a], 5[a]
School climate that provides little encouragement and support to students	4[a]
Lack of clear school policies regarding drug use	5[a]
Low teacher expectations of student achievement	5[a]
Low teacher and student morale	4[a]

Community/macro-level environment

Neighborhood disorganization	1, 2, 3, 5[a]
Low neighborhood attachment	1, 2, 3, 5[a]
Residential mobility/transitions and mobility/instability: transition and mobility	1, 2, 3,
High population density	3, 4[a]
Availability of alcohol and drugs	1, 2
Low community safety/high violence/high adult crime rates/ high rates of drug abuse	2, 3, 4[a], 5[a]

(continued)

Table 2.1 *(Continued)*

	Study Number (see below for reference)
Community regulation/laws favorable toward drug use, firearms, or crime	1, 2, 3, 5[a]
Pro-use messages specifically in advertising	5[a]
Negative community attitudes toward youth	2
Cultural norms about alcohol and drug use/community values and attitudes that are tolerant of substance abuse	3, 4[a], 5[a]
Hyperactivity	3
Lack of youth recreation opportunities/lack of cultural resources/lack of active community institutions	2, 3, 4[a]
Poverty and economic deprivation	1, 2, 3, 5[a]
Cultural disenfranchisement	5[a]
Situational/cultural factors	
Stressful events, multiple stressors, or both	2
High incidence of drug and alcohol use	2
Tension around cultural identity, acculturative stress, or both	2
Societal Factors	
National economic and employment conditions	5[a]
Discrimination	5[a]
Marginalization of groups	5[a]

[a] The authors also include several other demographic risk factors such as age, gender, race/ethnicity, socioeconomic status, employment, and education. Since these factors are not specified in a useful way, however, these factors are not presented here. For example, with this information only, which gender, male or female, is risk factor is uncertain.

Study introduced

(1)—1. Hawkins, J. D., Catalano, R. F., & Miller, J. Y. (1992). Risk and protective factors for alcohol and other drug problems in adolescence and early adulthood: Implications for substance abuse prevention. *Psychological Bulletin, 112*(1), 64–105.

(1)—2. Developmental Research and Programs. (1997). *Communities that care: Risk assessment for preventing adolescent problem behaviors.* Seattle, WA: Developmental Research and Programs.

(2) Holleran, L. K., Kim, Y., & Dixon, K. (2004). Innovative approaches to risk assessment within alcohol prevention programming. In A. R. Roberts & K. R. Yeager (Eds.), *Evidence-based practice manual: Research and outcome measures in health and human services* (pp. 677–684). New York: Oxford University Press.

(3) Jenson, J. M. (1997). Risk and protective factors for alcohol and other drug use in childhood and adolescence. In M. W. Fraser (Ed.), *Risk and resilience in childhood* (pp. 117–139). Washington, DC: NASW Press.

(4) National Institute on Drug Abuse. (1997). *Drug abuse prevention for at-risk groups* (NIH No. 97–4114). Rockville, MD: U.S. Department of Health and Human Services, National Institutes of Health.

(5) Brounstein, P. J., & Zweig, J. M. (1999). *Toward the 21st century: A primer on effective programs* (DHHS Publication No. [SMA]99–3301): Substance Abuse and Mental Health Services Administration.

studies that present risk factors for substance use/abuse, which range from individual attributes to macro-social environmental characteristics.

While risk factors increase the likelihood of problem incidence, protective factors reduce the likelihood because they buffer the impact of risk factors by augmenting strength. Complementing the risk factor model, prevention efforts based on a protective factor model focus on the positive and also modifiable factors rather than on less mutable risks such as temperament, genetic heritage, or low socioeconomic status. A major contribution of protective factor models to the prevention approach is that they shift the prevention paradigm from a psychopathological perspective to a healthy human development perspective (Holleran, Kim, & Dixon, 2004). According to 40 Developmental Assets of Search Institute (accessible at http://www.search-institute.org), one of the most widely used and effective protective factor models, protective factors can be classified into two categories, external assets and internal assets, with each category composed of 20 factors. The external and internal assets for elementary-age children are exhibited in the Table 2.2.

Other Characteristics of Selective Prevention

Targeting at-risk groups, selective prevention usually requires more intensive care, more professional skills, more varied treatment strategies, and a longer program duration compared to universal prevention (Kumpfer, 2003). The greatest merit of selective prevention lies in program efficiency and effectiveness. Despite larger program expenditure per capita, selective prevention is often considered more efficient than universal programs because it can cut down the total program cost by targeting individuals in need (NIDA, 1997a). In addition, a selective prevention approach can increase program efficiency by choosing optimum strategies that are well matched with identified risk factors of the program participants (Sullivan & Farrell, 2002). A particularly impressive facet of selective prevention is that its effect size is in general greater than that of universal prevention (Gottfredson & Wilson, 2003; Wilson, Gottfredson, & Najaka, 2001).

Selective prevention also has some limitations and practical difficulties. The biggest challenge in selective prevention is to identify and recruit at-risk group members. Even when a valid, precise, and reliable scale or screening instrument is available, serious weaknesses still remain. As selective prevention is directed toward at-risk subgroups of the general population, selective prevention inherently has a high possibility of stigmatization. Another limitation or difficulty of selective prevention approaches is that parents or family involvement, the core part of selective prevention, is not a simple job in practice, although a growing body of research notes that the parent component is essential for program success. At-risk populations often include poor families and single-parent families,

Table 2.2 Forty Developmental Assets for Elementary-Age Children

	External Assets		Internal Assets
Support	1. Family support 2. Positive family communication 3. Other adult relationships 4. Caring neighborhood 5. Caring out-of-home climate	Commitment to learning	21. Achievement expectation and motivation 22. Children are engaged in learning 23. Stimulating activity 24. Enjoyment of learning and bonding with school
Empowerment	6. Parent involvement in out-of-home situation 7. Community values children 8. Children are given useful roles 9. Service to others 10. Safety	Positive values	25. Reading for pleasure 26. Caring 27. Equality and social justice 28. Integrity 29. Honesty 30. Responsibility
Boundaries and expectations	11. Family boundaries 12. Out-of-home boundaries 13. Neighborhood boundaries 14. Adult role models 15. Positive peer observation 16. Appropriate expectations for growth	Social competencies	31. Healthy lifestyle and sexual attitudes 32. Planning and decision-making practice 33. Interpersonal skills 34. Cultural competence 35. Resistance skills 36. Peaceful conflict resolution
Constructive use of time	17. Creative activities 18. Out-of-home activities 19. Religious community 20. Positive, supervised time at home	Positive identity	37. Personal power 38. Self-esteem 39. Sense of purpose 40. Positive view of personal future

and many of these families do not have enough time or resources to ensure that the parents participate in and concentrate on the program.

What We Can Do

What Works? Effective Selective Prevention Programs for Elementary School Children

Although risk and protective models enhance prevention approaches, there are also some important warnings. Above all, it should be noticed that risk factors are not always causes of the problem (Fisher & Harrison, 2004). Rather, risks are correlates or covariates, which could be simple indicators or moderators of the problem (Pandina, 1996). This means that sometimes reducing the impact of risk factors does not necessarily decrease a student's substance use/abuse. This logic also applies to protective factors. Therefore, it is recommended that school social workers and other school-based practitioners examine successful programs, refer to research on program evaluation, and develop prevention strategies based on programs whose effectiveness is empirically proven. Although there is scant research that evaluates the effectiveness of selective prevention programs with rigorous scientific methods, there are some effective selective programs that can be considered model programs. Among those, selective prevention programs particularly appropriate for elementary school children are summarized in the Table 2.3.

Although all of these programs attempt to reduce the impact of risk factors and augment the effects of protective factors, they are different in terms of strength, limitations, program focus, and central strategies. Thus, it is suggested that professionals who envision substance use/abuse prevention programs scrutinize the primary resources and program strategies to select a best model program to utilize. If a model program is selected, a visit to the program Web site is recommended to glean useful information including program effectiveness, practitioner training, and economic costs of the program. Here, detailed information about the two selective prevention programs, SFP and PA program, are presented because these programs are considered particularly effective and applicable for elementary school settings.

The Strengthening Families Program

The SFP is a family skills training program designed to improve family life skills, parenting skills, and children's social skills (Kumpfer, Alvarado, & Whiteside, 2003). This program was developed by Karol Kumpfer and her associates in 1983, targeting elementary school–aged children who are at high risk for substance abuse and other problem behaviors. Over the last two decades, SFP has been revised and modified for different target populations such as junior high

Table 2.3 Effective Selective Preventions

Program and Duration	IOM	Target Population	Program Structure	Reported Effectiveness	Program Strategy
Across ages http://www.temple.edu/cil/Acrossaeshome.htm 1–3 yr.	Selective	9–13 yr. old	Intergenerational mentoring • Mentoring from qualified and trained elders • Life skills curriculum led by classroom teachers • Performing community service • Life/problem-solving curriculum • Workshop for parent and family members, which is designed to help them practice better parenting and participate in school activities	Quasi-experimental design research; the program showed desirable outcome in the follow ing areas: • Reactions to stress and anxiety • Self-perception • Attitudes toward school, elders, and future • Problem-solving skills/self-efficacy • Knowledge about substance use • Frequency of substance use	Primary strategy: • Community service • Mentoring • Community involvement Other strategies: • Personal/social competency • In-/after-school curricula • ATOD information dissemination • Peer resistance skill • Alternative activity • Family social/communication skills • Parenting/parent discipline • Parent–child interaction • Teacher involvement • Incentives for participation or completion

(continued)

Table 2.3 (Continued)

Program and Duration	IOM	Target Population	Program Structure	Reported Effectiveness	Program Strategy
CASASTART (Striving Together to Achieve Rewarding Tomorrows) http://www.casa columbia.org/absolutenm/templates/article.asp?articleid=287&zoneid=32 1–3 yr.	Selective Indicative	8–13 yr. old	• Case management that involves a home interview and monthly home visit • Academic support for children through tutoring and homework assistance • Social and emotional support for children through adult mentoring program • After-school curricular activities that includes recreational programs and trips • Community involvement that intends increased police presence and enhanced relationship among youth, families, and the police	Comparison of experimental subjects and control group at 1-year follow-up • Lower rate of past month use of any drugs, gateway drugs, & stronger drugs • Lower rate of past year use of any drugs and gateway drugs • Lower rate of lifetime use of any drugs or gateway drugs • Lower levels of violent crimes in the past year • Lower rate of involvement in drug sales during the past month • Lower rate of lifetime drug sales	Primary strategy: • Intensive case management • Family social/communication skills • Parenting/parent discipline Other strategies: • Academic support • In-/after-school curricula • ATOD information dissemination • Peer involvement • Alternative activity • Parent–child interaction • Parent–school relation • Community service • Mentoring • Community involvement • Incentives for participation or completion • Problem identification/referral

FAST (Families and Schools Together) http://www.wcer.wise.edu/fast/ 1–2 yr.	Universal Selective Indicative	5–14 yr. old	• Teacher identification of at-risk student • Outreach for program participants • Multifamily group sessions including parent–child play therapy (for 8 weeks) • Ongoing monthly reunions of the multifamily group (for 21 months)	• Decrease in anxiety-withdrawal of children • Increase in parent social support • Declines in attention problem and conduct disorder • Improved family cohesion • Long-term effect has been has been reported at 2–4 yr. follow-up • Program effectiveness appears consistent in more than 53 replication sites across the nation and Canada	Primary strategy: • Family social/communication skills • Parenting/parent discipline • Parent–child interaction Other strategies: • Personal/social competency • In-/after-school curricula • ATOD information dissemination • Peer resistance skill • Peer involvement • Alternative activity • Teacher involvement • Parent–school relation • Community involvement • Incentives for participation or completion

(continued)

Table 2.3 (Continued)

Program and Duration	IOM	Target Population	Program Structure	Reported Effectiveness	Program Strategy
Positive action http://www.posaction.com/ 0–12 yr.	Universal Selective Indicative	5–18 yr. old	• Daily classroom curriculum where teachers present 15- to 20-minute lessons (a total of 140 lessons) with various activities • School-climate program, which promotes the practice and reinforcement of schoolwide positive actions • Parent program that focuses on 42 weekly lessons for parents and encourages parent participation in school activities • Community program that is provided to community leaders so that a wide range of community service practices and cultivate positive actions within the community	• Program effectiveness has been observed in the following areas: academic achievement, absenteeism, discipline problem, violence and drug use, and criminal booking • Program effectiveness sustainedw in middle and high school years of the subjects • These outcome results have been replicated repeatedly	Primary strategy: • School reform • Teacher involvement • Parent–school relation Other strategies: • Personal/social competency • In-/after-school curricula • ATOD information dissemination • Peer resistance skill • Peer involvement • Family AOD Education • Community involvement

Projective achieve http://www.stopthinkachieve.com/ Over 3 yr.	Universal Selective	3–14 yr. old	• Stop & Think Social Skills program, in-school curricula that teach students desirable social and self-management skills • Parent training, tutoring, and support, which emphasizes ongoing parent–school collaboration • Effective classroom teacher/staff development, which is designed to increase their skills in strategic planning, organizational analysis, effective instructional and behavioral intervention • School reform, which intends more effective supports for social and academic development of students	• Decreased discipline referrals to the principal/the office • Improved in academic achievement • Decreased suspension & expulsion • Decreased grade retentions • Decreased special education referrals and placements	Primary strategy: • School reform • Teacher involvement Other strategies: • Personal/social competency • ATOD information dissemination • Peer resistance skill • Family social/ communication skills • Parenting/parent discipline • Parent–school relation • Community involvement

(continued)

Table 2.3 (*Continued*)

Program and Duration	IOM	Target population	Program Structure	Reported Effectiveness	Program Strategy
Strengthen families http://www. strengtheningfamiliesprogram.org 14–week courses	Universal Selective	6–12 yr. old	• Parent skills training that employs basic behavioral parent training techniques • Children's skills training designed to develop and enhance children's social and problem-solving skills • Family life skills training that utilizes family communication exercises • Two booster sessions at 6 and 12 months after the program, which encourage positive social networking	• Decreased use and intention to use ATOD among parents as well as children • Improved parent–child bonding, family relations, and communication • Improved children's academic achievement • Improved parents' discipline skills and parenting self-efficacy • Improved children's pro-social behaviors • Reduced children's problem behaviors including substance use • Reduced children's emotional problems including depression	Primary strategy: • Family social/ communication skills • Parenting/parent discipline • Parent–child interaction Other strategies: • Personal/social competency • Academic support • ATOD information dissemination • Peer resistance skill • Family AOD Education • Incentives for participation or completion

school students, preschool children, African Americans, and Hispanics/Latinos. SFP has shown significant effectiveness consistently in replications and various ethnic groups. For school social workers and other professionals who primarily work with elementary school children and their families, the original version of SFP program is introduced in this chapter.

Program Goal and Objectives

The ultimate goal of SFP is to enhance the resiliency of at-risk children. For this goal, SFP put primary focus on reduction of risk factors in family environment and enhancement of protective factors. Under this goal, SFP has three specified objectives and relevant strategies as follows (NIDA, 1997a, pp. 20–21):

- To increase parenting skills by
  increasing positive attention and praise
  increasing parents' levels of empathy for their children
  increasing parents' use of effective discipline
  decreasing parents' use of physical punishment
  decreasing parents' use of demonstrating use of substances
- To increase children's skills by
  increasing their communication skills
  increasing their skills to resist peer pressure to use substances
      or engage in other inappropriate behaviors
  increasing recognition of feelings
  increasing knowledge about alcohol and drugs
  increasing skills for coping with anger and criticism
  increasing compliance with parental requests
  increasing their self-esteem
  decreasing aggressive and other problem behaviors
  reducing intention to use in the future and the actual use
      of substances
- To improve family relationships by
  decreasing family conflicts
  improving family communications
  increasing parent–child time together
  increasing planning and organization skills

Target Population

The original SFP targets at-risk children 6 to 10 years of age whose parents are substance users or abusers. Since the original version of SPF demonstrated its effectiveness in the general child population as well as at-risk children, it can also be utilized as a universal prevention program.

Program Structure and Implementation

SFP program is composed of three primary components: parent skills training, children's skills training, and family skills training. The program participants have weekly sessions, each of which lasts 2 to 3 hours. The entire program continues for 14 consecutive weeks. For the first part of a weekly session, parents and children attend their own sessions separately. This is followed by a break, when snacks are served and announcements made. Then, the family skills training session starts, and the parents and children together practice the skills they learned in their own sessions. This format provides the participants with opportunities to learn their respective skills in their own sessions and then to practice the skills within the context of parent–child interaction. The entire program curricula for parent, children, and family skills training component are presented in the Table 2.4. As shown in the table, the topics of weekly sessions are coherent across groups so that family and children learn relevant skills at the same time and practice together.

Usually each parent skills training session starts with a review of homework and the concepts taught in the previous session. Then parents learn new concepts and skills. Finally, new homework relevant to the new concept and skills is assigned. The optimum group number for the parents' training session ranges from 8 to 12 with two skilled trainers. The basic format of the children's group session is similar to the parents'. The ideal group number is six to seven with two trainers. For smooth group work process and reinforcement of desirable behavior, children who follow group rules need to be rewarded with small prizes such as school supplies. The family training session is delivered in a format similar to that of the parents' or children's training session. Depending on the number of participants and accommodating capacity of the meeting place, family groups can be divided into several small groups or remain in one large group.

How to Implement Strengthening Families Program

Once a school chooses to use the SFP, a 2- to 3-day implementer training is conducted. A 415-page instructor manual contains a teaching outline, a script for the videotapes, and detailed instructions for all activities. Each lesson has an "overview" section providing practical considerations for successful implementation of SFP, such as a detailed timeline, list of equipments, master copies of worksheets, and homework assignments. A separate manual contains four booster sessions. There must be a teacher/facilitator for the parent session and the youth session, held concurrently. Cofacilitators are recommended where feasible. It is suggested that meals or snacks be included as incentives, and whenever possible, childcare and transportation should be provided.

Each child and parent session contains parallel content. They spend the first hour separately in separate skill-building sessions and then come together in supervised family activities. For example, while the children are learning about the importance of following rules, parents are working on enhancing their use

Table 2.4 Strengthen Families Program Curriculum

Week	Parent Skills Curriculum	Children Skills Curriculum	Family Skills Curriculum
1	Introduction and group building	Hello and rules	Introduction and group building
2	Developmental expectancies and stress management	Social skills I	Child's game I
3	Rewards	Social skills II	Child's game II: Rewards
4	Goals and objectives	Creating good behavior, secret rules of success	Child's game III: Goals and objectives
5	Differential attention/charts and spinners	How to say "NO" to stay out of trouble	Child's game IV: Differential attention/charts and spinners
6	Communication I	Communication I: Speaking and listening	Communication I: Speaking, listening, and coaching
7	Communication II	Communication II: Preparation for family meetings	Communication II: Family meetings
8	Alcohol, drugs, and families	Alcohol and drugs	Communication III: Learning from parents—parents' discussion
9	Problem-solving, giving directions	Problem-solving	Parents' game I: Problem-solving, giving directions
10	Limit setting I	Introduction to parents' game	Parents' game II: Consequences for noncompliance
11	Limit setting II	Coping skills I: Recognizing feelings	Parents' game III: Commands and time-out

(continued)

Table 2.4 (Continued)

Week	Parent Skills Curriculum	Children Skills Curriculum	Family Skills Curriculum
12	Limit setting III	Coping skills II: Dealing with criticism	Parent's game IV: Parent and child interaction on commands and consequences
13	Development/ implementation of behavior programs	Coping skills III: Coping with anger	Development/ implementation of family meetings and behavior change programs
14	Generalization and maintenance	Graduation, resources for help, and review	Graduation party

Source: From National Institute on Drug Absue (1997a).

of consequences when rules are broken; when the two groups combine in the family session, the children and family members practice problem solving with role-plays when a rule is followed or broken. The parent component has the following general goals: increase positive attention/praise, enhance empathy, teach supervision skills, decrease parents' drug use, increase positive modeling, and support the child's developmental stage. The family component provides a venue for children and families to practice and enhance listening, communication, respect, recognizing family strengths, cultural values, and effective problem-solving skills.

The groups utilize the following techniques: discussions, games, role-plays, activities, videotapes, and modeling of positive relationships and behaviors. The facilitator uses the videotapes, which include time countdowns for group discussions and activities. In fact, the facilitator starts the video as the session begins and lets it run for the full session to guide the curriculum and ensure staying on the task and accomplishment of session goals. Multiethnic video narrators conduct didactic presentations and are followed by family vignettes. Once the video is completed, the remaining time can be utilized for skill practice, discussions, and mutual support within the group.

Outcomes
Through extensive evaluation, the SFP has produced desirable outcomes and proved its effectiveness in various areas, including reduced use or intentions to use substances among children; reduced child problem behaviors, aggressiveness,

and emotional problems; decreased substance use among parents; improved parenting skills; and enhanced family communication skills. In a study that compared 71 SFP participating families with 47 nonparticipating families, for example, children of the SFP families were less likely to show behavioral, academic, social, and emotional problems than those of the non-SFP families (DeMarsh & Kumpfer, 1986). In addition, previously substance-using children as well as such parents showed significantly decreased use of tobacco and alcohol in pre- and posttest results (DeMarsh & Kumpfer, 1986).

Positive Action

Outlines
PA is a multifaceted program integrating classroom curriculum, schoolwide program, family component, and community-involvement components. Its primary goals include improvement of students' academic achievement, reduction of problem behaviors, and reinforcement of positive behaviors/attitudes. Primarily based on self-concept theories that emphasize actions rather than thoughts or feelings, PA attempts to teach students "what actions are positive, that they feel good when they do positive actions, and that they then have more positive thoughts and future actions" (Flay & Allred, 2003, p. S7). A major difference between PA and other selective prevention programs is that PA intends to affect more distal factors on student behavior in a holistic approach including school reorganization. The current PA program is the result of extensive pilot work and repeated evaluation that has been conducted since its first development by Carol Gerber Allred in 1977.

Program Goal and Objectives
PA has specified goals and objectives for the school and community as well as for the individual student and family (Flay, Allred, & Ordway, 2001, p. 76).
- Individual goals
  To give everyone the opportunity to learn and practice physical, intellectual, and emotional and social positive actions
  To understand that success and happiness means feeling good about who you are and what you are doing (being the best you can be)
  To develop good character, morals, and ethics
- Family goals
  To create a positive learning environment in the home
  To contribute to adult literacy and to develop life skills in adult family members
  To prepare children to be effective learners prior to entering school
- School goals
  To bring about comprehensive school reform

> To develop lifelong skills that lead to success and happiness in school and society
>
> To create a positive environment conducive to teaching and learning
>
> To create a safe, drug-free school environment
>
> To promote the personal and professional development of teachers, staff members, and administrators
>
> To completely unite the efforts of the school, home, and community organization in promoting the social, academic, and emotional growth of children
>
> To teach the leadership skills that will promote high achievement and expert performance in the global marketplace

- Community goals

> To involve the whole community in learning and practicing the positive actions necessary for a good self-concept and a successful life
>
> To contribute to a community environment

Target Population

PA targets children and adolescents 5 through 18 years of age. It can be implemented for the general student population as universal prevention, for at-risk students as selective prevention, and also for students with problem behaviors or mental health problems as indicated prevention.

Program Structure and Implementation

The PA program consists of a detailed classroom curriculum, a schoolwide climate program, and family- and community-involvement components. The classroom curriculum is composed of over 140 lessons. Guided by the teacher's kit, which includes a program manual for teachers and necessary materials, a classroom teacher presents a lesson for about 15–20 minutes almost every school day. This teacher-led classroom curriculum is delivered through various activities including stories, games, music, questions and answers, role-playing, posters, and manipulative activities. The classroom curriculum is organized in six units, which are presented in Table 2.5.

The school-climate program is designed to reinforce the practice of positive actions schoolwide. For this purpose, school administrators are encouraged to utilize various activities such as assemblies, celebrations, school newspaper, community service group for students, tutoring, and diversity initiatives. There is also a guiding manual for principals, the principal's kits. This principal's manual suggests utilizing stickers, tokens, and positive notes to reinforce positive actions of elementary school students. The parents' program has two major strategies, coordinated weekly lessons and strengthened connections between parent and school. With the purpose to help parents improve their communication skills and parenting style, the family kit introduces to parents 42 weekly lessons, which

Table 2.5 The Components of Positive Action Program

Unit/Number and Topic	Content
Unit 1. Self-concept: What it is, how it's formed, and why it's important	The relationship of thoughts, feelings, and actions (behavior). Units 2–6 teach children what actions are positive in various domains of life, that they feel good when they do positive actions, and that they then have more positive thoughts and future actions
Unit 2. Positive actions for body (physical) and mind (intellectual)	*Physical*: exercise, hygiene, nutrition, avoiding harmful substances, sleeping and resting enough, safety *Intellectual*: creative thinking, learning/studying, decision making, problem solving
Unit 3. Social/emotional positive actions for managing yourself responsibly	Manage human resources of time, energy, thoughts, actions, feelings (anger, fear, loneliness, others), talents, money, and possessions. Includes self-control
Unit 4. Social/emotional positive actions for getting along with others	Treat others the way you like to be treated, code of conduct (respect, fairness, kindness, honesty, courtesy, empathy, caring, responsible, reliable), conflict resolution, communication positively (communication skills), forming relationships, working cooperatively, community service. [These are the essence of character education]
Unit 5. Social/emotional positive actions for being honest with yourself & others	Self-honesty, doing what you will say you will do (integrity), not blaming others, not making excuses, not rationalizing; self-appraisal (look at strengths and weaknesses); and being in touch with reality. [These are the essence of mental health]
Unit 6. Social/emotional positive actions for improving yourself continually	Goal setting (physical, intellectual, and social/emotional), problem solving, decision making, believe in potential, have courage to try, turn problems into opportunities, persistence
Unit 7. Review	Review of all of above

Source: From Flay and Allred (2003, p. S8). Reproduced with permission.

are in coordination with the PA school curriculum and school-climate activities. In addition, parents are strongly encouraged to participate in various school activities, such as the decision-making team for the PA program, the development of the mission statement, and program evaluation procedures. The PA program also intends to create a better community environment that has a positive influence on child development. For this purpose, the community kit was developed. It provides community leaders, social service workers, public servants, and other stakeholders in the community with proper tools to promote positive actions, while playing their roles.

Outcomes

More than 7,000 schools have used the PA program nationally or internationally. The program has consistently showed desirable outcomes in case of substance use, absenteeism, disciplinary problems, violence, disruptive and disrespectful behaviors, school suspension, school dropout, and academic achievement including SAT scores, reading scores, and math scores. A recent study (Flay & Allred, 2003) evaluated the long-term effects of PA based on matched-school design. Below are the primary findings that show significant effects of the PA program on elementary school children:

- Students in PA schools performed 45% better, on average, in the Florida Reading Test than their counterparts in matched control schools.
- PA schools have 68% less violent incidents per 100 students compared to matched schools.
- The percentage of students who received out-of-school suspensions was 33.5% lower in PA schools as compared to matched schools.

Tools and Practice Examples

Through the several decades of experience in prevention of substance use/abuse, a substantial body of knowledge and skills has been accumulated. In the following sections, some of the critical information is summarized to guide school social workers and other professionals who are interested in at-risk children and preventive intervention programs.

What Needs to Be Done?

To be effective, school prevention programs should:

- *be based on the needs of students, families, school, and community.* The needs assessment will shed light on program focus by specifying the strengths and weaknesses of program participants and environment. Although assessment instruments should be chosen, the list of risk and protective factors can be utilized for a brief needs assessment.

- *have clear objectives.* Only when the goals and objectives are properly stated, the evaluation may produce reliable results. In addition, clear goals and objectives help practitioners keep the program focus and timelines (Knowles, 2001).
- *be based on comprehensive multidimensional perspective.* As seen earlier, risk and protective factors are situated at multisystem levels, indicating the necessity of a multidimensional approach in prevention efforts. This guideline has been supported by many empirical studies (e.g., St. Pierre et al., 2001; Tatchell, Waite, Tatchell, Durrant, & Bond, 2004).
- *focus on parent component.* Family involvement is the key for effective prevention (Gibson et al., 1993). Programs focusing on family relationships and parenting skills are usually effective in changing negative behaviors among parents as well as children (Gonet, 1994).
- *include competency skills.* Social competency models, such as life skills training, have shown desirable outcomes in various studies (Gonet, 1994), and the effectiveness has been validated for elementary school students (St. Pierre et al., 2001). A social competency component is considered appropriate for universal and selected prevention programs (Griffin, Botvin, Nichols, & Doyle, 2003).
- *utilize internal resources.* For young school children, as opposed to high school students, it is recommended that internal resources be utilized (e.g., teachers as implementers) rather than external resources (i.e., programs brought to the school by outside agencies) (Marsiglia, Holleran, & Jackson, 2000). Youth implementers, such as Peer Assistance and Leader (PAL) students, may be a great resource in elementary schools. Some of the assumptions about peer-led models, such as the fear of control and discipline difficulties, are unfounded (Erhard, 1999). It is also important to note that, in the sensitive area of substance use and abuse, peer-led programs yielded twice as much participants' self-disclosure (Erhard, 1999). All in all, there are strong indications that peer-led models may possess great potential for prevention efforts.
- *be delivered in interactive method.* Compared to a noninteractive method, an interactive method produces greater effect size (Tobler, 1992). In some cases, a program showed effectiveness only when delivered in an interaction method (Sussman, Rohrbach, Ratel, & Holiday, 2003).
- *be implemented in an intended way.* Well-developed and empirically proven prevention models usually have specified program manuals. To achieve program effectiveness, high fidelity is a must (Hogan, Gabrielsen, Luna, & Grothaus, 2003).
- *be followed by a booster program.* It is always recommended to provide booster sessions after program completion as the booster programs are

vital for long-lasting program effectiveness (Gottfredson & Wilson, 2003; Lilja, Wilhelmsen, Larsson, & Hamilton, 2003).

What Should Be Avoided?

To be effective, school prevention programs should:

- *not target individuals with a substance abuse problem.* Only qualified specialists on drug use should provide intervention programs to identified substance users or abusers. If school social workers and counselors (given that they are not drug abuse specialists) find a student who needs intervention, they must refer the student to a proper clinical setting (Gibson et al., 1993).
- *not just provide information.* Information or knowledge on substance use/abuse does not necessarily reduce substance use (Holleran et al., 2004; Petosa, 1992; Stoil & Hill, 1996). In the worst cases, it could increase substance use among children or adolescents (Gonet, 1994).
- *not threaten students.* Persuading children not to use a substance in a threatening way is not effective. Rather, it could cause mistrust toward mental health professions (Gonet, 1994).
- *not be completed in a one-shot program.* A one-shot program, such as a guest speaker or film-watching, is usually least effective (Gonet, 1994).
- *not use a self-esteem component as a primary strategy.* Programs that focus on self-esteem have not been the most effective. Program results in such models are not consistent and too often disappointing (Stoil & Hill, 1996).

Key Points to Remember

In this chapter, the authors presented an overview of selective prevention interventions, explained a risk and protective factor paradigm, and provided two examples of evidence-based model programs, the SFP and PA. It closes with critical recommendations and practical guidelines for utilizing such interventions. As with any program, and especially with elementary school students, practitioners must be very careful to protect the confidentiality of students and families. In addition, when doing prevention interventions with children, it is vital that clinicians avoid labeling and stereotyping. It is helpful to recognize that interventions that address substance abuse prevention, as noted previously, also prevent other problematic outcomes, such as rebelliousness, aggression, and absenteeism. It is also recommended that teachers and program implementers watch students carefully for potential negative responses to the intervention (e.g., emotional overload, anxiety, and depression), which might give clues that other concurrent issues or more serious problems exist. In such cases, referral to a specialist or a proper clinical setting may be necessary.

3 Screening Substance Use/Abuse of Middle and High School Students

Lori K. Holleran

Soyon Jung

Getting Started

Adolescent substance use has been a major concern in this country. According to the Monitoring the Future (MTF) study conducted by the University of Michigan (University of Michigan Institute for Social Research, 2003) and supported by the National Institute on Drug Abuse (NIDA), a high percentage of American youth has tried or currently use various illicit drugs, alcohol, and tobacco. Among the 8th, 10th, and 12th graders surveyed in 2003, for example, one third were using alcohol and one sixth smoked cigarettes. In addition, many adolescents use illegal drugs including marijuana, ecstasy, and LSD. Approximately 17% reported illicit drug use during the month prior to the survey and 37% reported that they had tried it at least once during their lifetime.

The consequences of substance use are serious, costly, and extensive. Most substances have immediate physiological influences. They interfere with correct perception and rational judgment (McWhirter, McWhirter, McWhirter, & McWhirter, 2004). It is well established that adolescents are more likely to be involved in risk-taking behaviors under the influence of substance(s). Not surprisingly, substance use often leads to fatal accidents and crime. Alcohol consumption, for instance, is a major cause of death among youth via motor vehicle accidents, homicides, suicides, and drowning (U.S. Department of Health and Human Services [DHHS], 2000). Furthermore, heavy drinking and smoking often contribute to various diseases: cancer, heart disease, many liver-related diseases (DHHS, 2000), and sexually transmitted diseases, including HIV/AIDS (Centers for Disease Control and Prevention, 2004). The economic costs of substance abuse and drug abuse in the United States were estimated to be $167 and $110 billion, respectively, in 1995 (DHHS, 2000). Substance use has detrimental impacts on the mental health of adolescents as well. Newcomb and Bentler (1989) found that serious drug users are vulnerable to experience loneliness, depression, and suicide ideations. Moreover, substance use hinders youth from accomplishing important developmental tasks, performing expected duties, and building healthy relationships with others. Previous studies have consistently indicated that substance use is significantly associated with poor educational outcomes and academic failure (Jeynes, 2002; NCCDPHP, 2000;

43

National Commission on Drug-Free Schools, 1990), physical fights and criminal behavior (NCCDPHP, 2000), and inadequate positive social connection (Havighurst, 1972).

Although the detrimental consequences of adolescent substance use are immense, appropriate treatment can significantly reduce the harmful effects (Winters, Latimer, & Stinchfield, 1999). Early intervention is considered especially desirable in terms of effectiveness and efficiency. The Consensus Panel for the Center for Substance Abuse Treatment (CSAT) recommends that all adolescents showing any sign of substance use be properly screened (Winters, 2001b). Thus, professionals who work with at-risk youth must have screening resources and expertise so that the adolescents can receive more comprehensive assessment and intervention services (Winters, 2001b). Because adolescents spend a large amount of time at school, the role of school mental health professionals in identifying substance users at earlier stages and providing them with intervention opportunities cannot be overemphasized.

This chapter discusses the substance use/abuse screening methods that school mental health professionals can easily utilize. A summary table of screening tools developed particularly for the adolescent population is presented. Somewhat detailed information about two screening instruments, Problem-Oriented Screening Instruments for Teenagers (POSIT) and Rutgers Alcohol Problem Index (RAPI), which are considered most efficient at school settings, follows. This information covers how to administer the instruments and how to interpret the results. Finally, a case example is provided to demonstrate the techniques described in the chapter.

Substance users need to be aware of their problems and motivated for change with regard to substances during each screening procedure (Winters, 2001b). School mental health professionals should remember to utilize their most astute clinical techniques to make successful initial contacts with potential substance users and refer them to suitable intervention programs.

What We Know and Can Do

Screening Adolescent Substance Use/Abuse

Before examining specific screening methods and procedures, it is necessary to understand the differences between screening, assessment, and diagnosis of substance use/abuse. The primary purpose of screening is to identify potential substance users who need a through assessment (Winters, 2001b). On the other hand, comprehensive assessment aims to verify substance use/abuse of an adolescent and reveal other relevant problems and service needs (Winters, 2001b). Diagnosis is carried out on the basis of the most comprehensive measures or highly structured criteria such as those presented in the fourth edition of the *Diagnostic and Statistical Manual of Mental Disorders* (*DSM-IV*). Diagnosis is considered a more decisive conclusion compared to assessment. While *assessment* refers to "the process of gathering information," *diagnosis* is defined as the "the conclusion that is reached on the basis of the assessment" (Fisher & Harrison, 2004, p. 84).

One important point that school mental health professionals should keep in mind is that a comprehensive substance use/abuse assessment or diagnosis is best conducted by alcohol, tobacco, and other drug (commonly referred to as ATOD) specialists in general, and those involved in the intervention plan or treatment service in particular. Thus, it is recommended for school mental health professionals to provide screening services only, unless they have adequate qualification for substance use/abuse assessment and diagnosis (Fisher & Harrison, 2004).

Who Needs to Be Screened?

Because substance use is quite prevalent among American youth and many of them are diverge from the stereotypes of ATOD users, school social workers and school counselors need to be always aware that the possibility of a substance use problem exists when they are providing any kind of service to students. Ideally, screenings for substance use/abuse should be done universally with all students. However, given limited resources and inadequate numbers of mental health professionals at school, it would be more desirable to focus on screening students at risk for substance use/abuse or showing some indication of possible substance use.

An effective way to identify potential substance users for screening is to utilize a multidisciplinary team including classroom teachers. Because classroom teachers spend much time with students and have many opportunities to observe student behaviors directly, they can make a significant contribution to problem identification (Gonet, 1994). School social workers and drug counselors can encourage participation of teachers in case identification procedures and enhance the quality of information reported by the teachers, using a form specially designed to easily detect substance use among students.

Self-Report Screening Instruments for Adolescents

Although there are various approaches available, self-report screening instruments are commonly used to identify ATOD problem among adolescents (Martin & Winters, 1998). Using standardized instruments has some advantages: it reduces potential bias (Winters, 2001a); it is less likely to threaten students than other methods (Winters, 2001a); and it makes mental health professionals look trustworthy (Orenstein, Davis, & Wolfe, 1995). If school mental health professionals plan to use self-report screening instruments, the biggest challenge is selecting the best instrument for a given situation. Fortunately, many screening instruments for the adolescent population have been developed in recent years and now there is a wide range of appropriate instruments. Table 3.1 briefly introduces nine screening instruments for adolescents suitable for school settings. Because the characteristics of the instruments are very diverse, school mental health professions are advised to check the qualities, cost, and required conditions of the instruments thoroughly before choosing one. Among the nine

Table 3.1 Screening Instruments for Adolescent Substance or Alcohol Use/Abuse

Name of Screening Tool and Contact Info for Access:
Adolescent Alcohol Involvement Scale (AAIS)
http://www.niaaa.nih.gov/publications/aais.htm

Brief Description:
- Problems measured: alcohol use and psychosocial consequences
- Administration: self-report
- Required qualification for use: no specific requirement
- Reliability: test–retest and internal consistency
- Validity: construct and criterion (predictive, concurrent, postdictive)

Number of Q (time):
14 (5 m)

Reading Level:
No information

Cost[a] and Copyright:
Cost information is not available
Copyright status is unknown

Key Reference:
Mayer and Filstead (1979)

Name of Screening Tool and Contact Info for Access:
Adolescent Drinking Index (ADI)
Psychological Assessment Resources, Inc.
PO Box 998, Odessa, FL 33556 (800) 331–8378
http://www.parinc.com/index.cfm

Brief Description:
- Problems measured: severity of drinking problems
- Administration: self-report or interview
- Qualification for administration: (1) a bachelor's degree or higher in psychology or a related field; or (2) adequate training for interpreting psychological test results
- Reliability: internal consistency
- Validity: criterion (concurrent validity)

(continued)

Table 3.1 *(Continued)*

Number of Q (time):
24 (5 m)

Reading Level:
5th grade

Cost[a] and Copyright:
Introductory kit: $82
Professional manual: $35
Test booklets (pkg/25): $53

Key Reference:
Mental Measurements Yearbook (12th ed.)

Name of Screening Tool and Contact Info for Access:
Adolescent Drug Involvement Scale (ADIS)
D. Paul Moberg, Ph.D.
Center for Health Policy & Program Evaluation
Univ. of Wisconsin at Madison
2710 Marshall Ct., Madison, WI 53705
(608) 263–1304

Brief Description:
• Problems measured: levels of drug use other than alcohol
• Administration: self-report
• Qualification for administration: no specific requirement
• Reliability: internal consistency
• Validity: criterion (concurrent)

Number of Q (time):
12 (4–5 m)

Reading Level:
No information

Cost[a] and Copyright:
No cost
ADIS is in public domain

Key Reference:
Moberg and Hahn (1991)

Name of Screening Tool and Contact Info for Access:
CRAFFT[b]
American Medical Association
Licensing and Permission
515 N. State Street
Chicago, IL 60610

Brief Description:
• Problems measured: substance use problem
• Administration: self-report

(continued)

47

Table 3.1 (Continued)

- Required qualification for use: no information available
- Reliability: internal consistency
- Validity: criterion

Number of Q (time):
6

Reading Level:
No information

Cost[a] and Copyright:
No cost
Copyrighted

Key Reference:
Knight, Shrier, Bravender, Farrell, Bilt, and Shaffer (1999)

Name of Screening Tool and Contact Info for Access:
Drug and Alcohol Problem (DAP) Quick Screen
Richard H. Schwartz, M.D.
410 Maple Avenue West
Vienna, VA 22180
(703) 338–2244

Brief Description:
- Problems measured: overall problem of alcohol and other drug use
- Administration: self-report or interview
- Qualification for administration: no specific requirement
- Reliability and validity: this scale has been tested in a pediatric practice setting. However, reliability and validity of the DAP Quick Screen have not been evaluated

Number of Q (time):
30 (10 m)

Reading Level:
6th grade

Cost[a] and Copyright:
No cost
DAP is in public domain

Key Reference:
Schwartz and Wirtz (1990)

Name of Screening Tool and Contact Info for Access:
Drug Use Screening Inventory Revised (DUSI-R)[c]
The Gordian Group
P.O. Box 1587
Hartsville, SC 29950
(843) 383–2201
www.dusi.com

(continued)

Table 3.1 *(Continued)*

Brief Description:
- Problems measured: severity of disturbance in 10 domains including drug and alcohol use, substance use, behavior patterns, and health status.
- Administration: self-report
- Qualification for administration: drug counselors and other qualified users
- Reliability and validity: good levels of reliability and validity of DUSI-R have been reported

Number of Q (time):
159 (20–40 m)

Reading Level:
5th grade

Cost^a and Copyright:
A copy of paper
DUSI-R: $2
DUSI-R software for computer administration: $199

Copyrighted

Key Reference:
Kirisci, Mezzich, and Tarter (1995)

Name of Screening Tool and Contact Info for Access:
Personal Experience Screening Questionnaire (PESQ)
Western Psychological Services
12031 Wilshire Blvd.
Los Angeles, CA 90025
(310) 478–2061
http://www.wpspublish.com/Inetpub4/index.htm

Brief Description:
- Problems measured: problem severity, psychosocial items, and drug use history
- Administration: self-report or interview
- Qualification for administration: no specific requirement
- Reliability: internal consistency
- Validity: content, construct, and criterion (postdictive and concurrent)

Number of Q (time):
40 (10 m)

Reading Level:
No information

Cost^a and Copyright:
$79.50 per kit (each kit includes 25 Autoscore Test Forms and 1 Manual)

Copyrighted

Key Reference:
Winters (1991), Winters (1992)

(continued)

Table 3.1 *(Continued)*

Name of Screening Tool and Contact Info for Access:
Problem-Oriented Screening Instrument for Teenagers (POSIT)[b]
Elizabeth Rahdert, Ph.D.
National Institute on Drug Abuse, NIH
5600 Fishers Lane, Room 10A-10
Rockville, MD 20857
(301) 443-0107

Brief Description:
- Goal: to identify substance abuse and related problems and to estimate potential service needs in 10 system areas
- Type: paper-and-pencil questionnaire CD-ROM version is also available
- Administration: self-report or interview
- Qualification for administration: no specific requirement
- Reliability: test–retest and internal consistency
- Validity: content, criterion (concurrent & predictive), construct validity (convergent & discriminant)

Number of Q (time):
139 (20–30 m)

Reading Level:
5th grade (12–19 yr old)

Cost[a] and Copyright:
No cost
POSIT is in public domain

Key Reference:
Rahdert (1991)

Name of Screening Tool and Contact Info for Access:
Rutgers Alcohol Problem Index (RAPI)
Helene Raskin White, Ph.D.
Center of Alcohol Studies
Rutgers University
P.O. Box 969
Piscataway, NJ 08855–0969
(732) 445–3579

Brief Description:
- Problems assessed: problem drinking of adolescents
- Administration: self-report or interview
- Qualification for administration: no training required
- Reliability: split-half, internal consistency
- Validity: content and criterion
- RAPI is appropriate for use in clinical and nonclinical samples of adolescents and young adults

(continued)

Table 3.1 *(Continued)*

Number of Q (time):
23 (10 m)

Reading Level:
7th grade

Cost[a] and Copyright:
No cost
Copyrighted

Key Reference:
White and Labouvie (1989)

---

[a] Cost as of July, 2004.
[b] CRAFFT questions can be obtained from http://www.slp3d2.com/rwj_1027/webcast/docs/
screentest.html
[c] Indicates that Spanish version is available.

---

instruments, POSIT and RAPI are especially recommendable for school mental health professionals considering their low cost, copyright, easy access, and psychometric traits. Thus, these instruments are presented as exemplars.

Problem-Oriented Screening Instrument for Teenagers

Brief Description

POSIT is one of the most widely used instruments for adolescent substance use/abuse.[1] It was developed by NIDA to identify the potential problems and service needs of adolescents aged 12 to 19 years. It is composed of 139 Yes/No questions under the following 10 subscales: Substance Use and Abuse; Physical Health Status; Mental Health Status; Family Relations; Peer Relations; Educational Status; Vocational Status; Social Skills; Leisure and Recreation; and Aggressive Behavior and Delinquency.

Format and Administration

The original POSIT is a paper-and-pencil questionnaire. A CD-ROM version is also available. It can be self-administered or administered during an interview in a variety of settings including schools. No specific qualification is necessary for administration.

Scoring and Interpretation

POSIT can be scored and interpreted in two different ways, using either the original or the new scoring system. In the original scoring system, the questions are classified as general, age-related, or red-flag items. While every point-earning answer to general items adds one risk score in each subscale, the answer to age-related items applies only to the teenagers in a specified age range. Either any point earning in red-flag items or expert-based cutoff score in a subscale is interpreted as indication of needs for further assessment or service in the problem area. In a new scoring system, however, red-flag items are not taken into account and the total score of each subscale is used to determine the level of risks in the area.

Psychometric Properties

The internal consistency of POSIT varies across the subscales and different studies. Some subscales, such as Substance Use/Abuse, Mental Health, and Aggressive Behavior/Delinquency, exhibit high levels of internal consistency, whereas others, such as Leisure/Recreation, Vocational Status, and Physical Health, show lower levels of internal consistency than conventionally acceptable ranges. However, it should be noticed that the Cronbach's alpha for the Substance Use/Abuse subscale has been identified as high, ranging from .77 (Knight, Goodman, Pulerwitz, & DuRant, 2001) to .93 (Melchior, Rahdert, & Huba, 1994). Acceptable levels of test–retest reliability have also been reported (Dembo, Schmeidler, & Henly, 1996; McLaney & Boca, 1994). All the subscales of POSIT have successfully differentiated heavy substance users from nonusers, showing good concurrent differential validity (Melchior et al., 1994). In a study (McLaney & Boca, 1994) in which POSIT was compared with Personal Experience Inventory (PEI), Diagnostic Interview for Children and Adolescents (DICA), and the Adolescent Diagnostic Interview (ADI), POSIT also showed both convergent and divergent validity.

Brief Evaluation of the Instrument

Based on earlier empirical studies, POSIT is a recommendable screening instrument especially for substance use/abuse problems among adolescents. One of the advantages of POSIT lies in its comprehensiveness. The screening results with POSIT can identify potential problems in various areas rather than assessing substance use problems only. Such comprehensiveness might help mental health professionals make better referrals for further assessment or necessary services based on various needs of the adolescents. Easy administration and cost-effectiveness are also the considerable benefits of using POSIT. In addition, POSIT is in the public domain and can be easily obtained at no cost by contacting NIDA or the National Clearinghouse for Alcohol and Drug Information, or by visiting the Web site of the National Institute on Alcohol Abuse and Alcoholism.

Rutgers Alcohol Problem Index

Brief Description

RAPI is a simple, unidimensional screening tool for problem drinking. Its target populations are adolescents and young adults aged 12 to 21 years. The researchers at the Center of Alcohol Studies, Rutgers University, developed RAPI in

1989 to create an efficient and conceptually sound instrument to assess problem drinking among adolescents. This instrument has been validated on nonclinical as well as clinical samples.

Format and Administration

RAPI is composed of 23 items describing alcohol-related problems or symptoms. The original version of RAPI asks respondents how many times they experienced each problem during the last 3 years, and provides five answer categories for each question: none; 1–2 times; 3–4 times; 6–10 times; and more than 10 times. A later version of RAPI[2] asks respondents the same questions, but the time frame was reduced to the previous year alone for greater specificity, as shown in Table 3.2. The number of answer categories was also reduced to four, ranging from "none" to "more than five times." Basically, RAPI is a self-administered paper-and-pencil type instrument, but it can also be easily administered in an interview format if preferable or necessary. No special training is required for administration.

Table 3.2 Rutgers Alcohol Problem Index (RAPI)

Different things happen to people while they are drinking ALCOHOL or because of *ALCOHOL* drinking. Several of these things are listed below. Indicate how many times each of these things happened to you WITHIN THE LAST YEAR.

Use the following code:
0 = None
1 = 1–2 times
2 = 3–5 times
3 = More than 5 times

None	1–2 Times	3–5 Times	More Than 5 Times	HOW MANY TIMES HAS THIS HAPPENED TO YOU WHILE YOU WERE DRINKING OR BECAUSE OF YOUR DRINKING DURING THE LAST YEAR?
0	1	2	3	Not able to do your homework or study for a test
0	1	2	3	Got into fights with other people (friends, relatives, strangers)
0	1	2	3	Missed out on other things because you spent too much money on alcohol
0	1	2	3	Went to work or school high or drunk

(continued)

Table 3.2 (Continued)

None	1–2 Times	3–5 Times	More Than 5 Times	HOW MANY TIMES HAS THIS HAPPENED TO YOU WHILE YOU WERE DRINKING OR BECAUSE OF YOUR DRINKING DURING THE LAST YEAR?
0	1	2	3	Caused shame or embarrassment to someone
0	1	2	3	Neglected your responsibilities
0	1	2	3	Relatives avoided you
0	1	2	3	Felt that you needed *more* alcohol than you used to in order to get the same effect
0	1	2	3	Tried to control your drinking (tried to drink only at certain times of the day or in certain places, that is, tried to change your pattern of drinking)
0	1	2	3	Had withdrawal symptoms, that is, felt sick because you stopped or cut down on drinking
0	1	2	3	Noticed a change in your responsibility
0	1	2	3	Felt that you had a problem with alcohol
0	1	2	3	Missed a day (or part of a day) of school or work
0	1	2	3	Wanted to stop drinking but couldn't
0	1	2	3	Suddenly found yourself in a place that you could not remember getting to
0	1	2	3	Passed out or fainted suddenly
0	1	2	3	Had a fight, argument, or bad feeling with a friend
0	1	2	3	Had a fight, argument, or bad feeling with a family member

(continued)

Table 3.2 (Continued)

None	1–2 Times	3–5 Times	More Than 5 Times	HOW MANY TIMES HAS THIS HAPPENED TO YOU WHILE YOU WERE DRINKING OR BECAUSE OF YOUR DRINKING DURING THE LAST YEAR?
0	1	2	3	Kept drinking when you promised yourself not to
0	1	2	3	Felt you were going crazy
0	1	2	3	Had a bad time
0	1	2	3	Felt physically or psychologically dependent on alcohol
0	1	2	3	Was told by a friend, neighbor, or relative to stop or cut down drinking

Scoring and Interpretation

Scoring of RAPI is simple. If the number assigned to each answer category is added, it forms a total scale score. It should be noted, however, that the last two answer categories of the original version of RAPI need to be combined and three be assigned. Therefore, the total scores of both the original and later version of RAPI range from 0 to 69. The total score is considered to be an indicator of the level of problem drinking. The necessity for a further assessment can be made based on the norms available. According to recent data provided by the RAPI developers, the mean scores for clinical sample range from 21 to 26, while those for nonclinical sample from 5.9 to 8.2, depending on gender and age. Specific information about RAPI mean score is exhibited in Table 3.3.

Psychometric Properties

The 23-item RAPI resulted from factor analyses conducted on a nonclinical sample of 1,308 adolescents (White & Labouvie, 1989). Its internal consistency measured was .92 and test–retest with a 3-year period marked .40 (White & Labouvie, 1989). RAPI has showed high correlation levels with Adolescent Alcohol Involvement Scale (AAIS), Alcohol Dependence Scale (ADS), DSM-III, and DSM-III-R (greater than .70), indicating good convergent validity. In addition, RAPI can differentiate seriously problematic drinkers from non- or less problematic drinkers in adolescence.

Table 3.3 Currently Available Mean Scores of RAPI					
Clinical Sample	N	Mean	Nonclinical Sample	N	Mean
14–16-year-old males	42	23.3	14–16-year-old males	151	7.5
14–16-year-old females	19	22.2	14–16-year-old females	147	5.9
17–18-year-old males	43	21.1	17–18-year-old males	211	8.2
17–18-year-old females	15	26.0	17–18-year-old females	208	7.4

Brief Evaluation of the Instrument

As a screening instrument for adolescents, RAPI has several merits. First, it is efficient. Its administration and scoring procedures are simple and require only 15 minutes or less (10 minutes for administration and 3 to 5 minutes for scoring). It is in the public domain, and no cost is involved. Second, RAPI has high utility. It can be used for nonclinical as well as clinical samples. Third, all the RAPI items are worded appropriately for teenage students and are easy to understand. Fourth, it can be used for various purposes. Based on RAPI scores, for example, service referral can be done properly and the effectiveness of the intervention program for adolescent drinkers can be evaluated. Furthermore, according to the scale developers, it is possible to use RAPI to assess all types of substance use problems. The only thing necessary is to use proper words for the substance instead of "alcohol" or "drinking." RAPI has also some limitations. Most notably, there is no clear cutoff point based on which adolescents with a drinking problem and adolescents without a problem can be classified. Another limitation is that RAPI measures only one problem area (e.g., alcohol use/abuse). Considering previous studies that have consistently found that substance use/abuse problems are complicated and related to many other areas, it would be more desirable to use RAPI with other instruments for more accurate screening or comprehensive assessment.

Tools and Practice Examples

Tools

The student behavior checklist, which is composed of the indicative signs of substance use/abuse and relevant problem behaviors as shown in Figure 3.1, is a good example of a tool used to screen for substance use. School mental health professionals can ask teachers to fill out this form and submit it to the interdisciplinary team or the professionals whenever the teachers find a potential substance user.

Teacher Name:--------------   Date:--------

_____ (student name) has been referred to the "CARE" team. Please help us by sharing information about his or her school behavior. This information will be strictly confidential. Thank you for your cooperation.

Check those behaviors you have witnessed. Use the bottom of this form if you have any further information that you think may be of help to the CARE team. Thank you.

_____ Tardy:	No. _____	_____ Nonresponsiveness
_____ Absent:	No. _____	_____ Lack of motivation

Frequent requests to go to:

_____ Lav.	_____ Phone	_____ Defensiveness
_____ Clinic	_____ Counselor	_____ Withdrawn; loner
Other (specify) _____		_____ Erratic behavior from day to day
_____ Falling asleep		_____ Cheating
_____ Slurred speech		_____ Constantly in "wrong" area
_____ Incoherent		(specify)_____
_____ Stumbles		_____ Obscene language or gestures
Smells of:		_____ Dramatic attention-getting behavior
_____ Alcohol	_____ Mouthwash	_____ Sudden outbursts
_____ Cigarette Smoke	_____ Marijuana	_____ Verbal abuse
_____ Talk freely of drug/alcohol use		_____ Fighting
_____ Brown-stained fingertips		_____ Class interruptions for this student
_____ Bad hygiene		_____ Change of friends (negative)
_____ Unusual/frequent bruises or sores		_____ Frequent requests for schedule changes
_____ Declining grade(s)		_____ Poor work performance
From _____ to _____		
_____ Other unacceptable out-of-class behavior		_____ Other unacceptable out-of-class behavior
Example:_____		Example:_____

Use this space for any other pertinent comments:_____

Please deposit this from in an envelope in the CARE Mailbox in the Main Office.

Figure 3.1. A Sample Behavioral Checklist.

Source: From *Counseling the Adolescent substance Abuser: School-Based Intervention and Prevention* (p. 93), by M. M. Gonet, 1994, Thousand Oaks, CA: Sage. Reprinted with Permission.

Case Example

Phil is a 15-year-old male whose behavior has recently changed dramatically. He has a history of being a strong student with aspirations to attend college and write creatively. He had always been somewhat eccentric, dressing uniquely, with unusual hairdos, but recently appeared disheveled and unkempt. Upon noticing an undeniable drop in his grades and motivation, his English teacher utilized the student behavior checklist, particularly noting the following behaviors: excessive tardiness, frequent requests to go to the restroom, cell phone buzzing throughout class, moments of apparent disorientation, noticeable chewing of breath mints in succession, occasionally nodding off in class. When the teacher requested a meeting with Phil, she noticed that his breath smelled of alcohol. Having a strong relationship with Phil in the past, she expressed concern and requested that he meet with her to talk. She kept her comments to factual observations rather than emotional and speculative responses. She framed her interactions in empathy and supportively suggested that they invite the school social worker to talk. Phil refused initially, but with warm encouragement and strength-based, positive persuasion, he agreed to meet with the worker.

Prior to the screening, a multidisciplinary team consisting of the school social worker, classroom teachers, specialty teachers (e.g., P.E. and art), the school nurse, and principal were made aware of concerns about Phil by his English teacher. The teacher had suggested that Phil's recent change in attention span would make in-depth screening difficult, and the team and social worker decided to begin with the RAPI.

The social worker began by noting very specific strengths of the student (i.e., his aptitude for writing, his history of good grades, his bold sense of style, and his sense of humor) and then gently noted the shifts that the teacher had recognized. She cleverly described that alcohol use and experimentation are common in his age-group. Further, she persuaded Phil to understand that she needed to learn more about his drinking since the teacher's concerns included awareness that he drank occasionally. She also started by asking if he had any friend who drank, because the associations that one has provides a good clue on habits. He openly noted that a few of his friends liked to drink, but that he only did it "once in a while." Sensing his hesitancy, she clearly described that their discussion would remain confidential, except for if the information denoted danger to self or others. She stated that she would start by conducting a brief questionnaire to get a general sense of the issues. She encouraged him to be open and honest and to ask questions if he had any. She added that she would do her best to help and advocate for the student, and that she could be most effective if he was as honest as possible. This gave him the sense that she was trying to help rather than trap or punish him. She handed him the RAPI, and he scored on the items shown in Table 3.4.

None	1–2 Times	3–5 Times	More Than 5 Times	HOW MANY TIMES HAS THIS HAPPENED TO YOU WHILE YOU WERE DRINKING OR BECAUSE OF YOUR DRINKING DURING THE LAST YEAR?
0	1	X	3	Not able to do your homework or study for a test
0	X	2	3	Got into fights with other people (friends, relatives, strangers)
X	1	2	3	Missed out on other things because you spent too much money on alcohol
0	X	2	3	Went to work or school high or drunk
X	1	2	3	Caused shame or embarrassment to someone
0	X	2	3	Neglected your responsibilities
0	1	X	3	Relatives avoided you
X	1	2	3	Felt that you needed more alcohol than you used to in order to get the same effect
X	1	2	3	Tried to control your drinking (tried to drink only at certain times of the day or in certain places, that is, tried to change your pattern of drinking)
X	1	2	3	Had withdrawal symptoms, that is, felt sick because you stopped or cut down on drinking
0	1	X	3	Noticed a change in your responsibility
X	1	2	3	Felt that you had a problem with alcohol
0	1	2	X	Missed a day (or part of a day) of school or work
X	1	2	3	Wanted to stop drinking but couldn't

Table 3.4 Phil's RAPI Test Result

(continued)

Table 3.4 (Continued)

None	1–2 Times	3–5 Times	More Than 5 Times	HOW MANY TIMES HAS THIS HAPPENED TO YOU WHILE YOU WERE DRINKING OR BECAUSE OF YOUR DRINKING DURING THE LAST YEAR?
X	1	2	3	Suddenly found yourself in a place that you could not remember getting to
X	1	2	3	Passed out or fainted suddenly
0	X	2	3	Had a fight, argument or bad feeling with a friend
X	1	2	3	Kept drinking when you promised yourself not to
0	1	2	X	Felt you were going crazy
0	1	2	X	Had a bad time
X	1	2	3	Felt physically or psychologically dependent on alcohol
0	1	2	X	Was told by a friend, neighbor or relative to stop or cut down drinking

Phil's answers clearly showed a lack of concern about his own alcohol use and a belief that he could stop at any time. However, he had admitted that alcohol had played a role in affecting his academic work, family relationships, and peer relationships (he specifically commented that his girlfriend didn't drink or smoke "pot" and was thinking of breaking up with him if he did). The social worker reviewed his responses and shared his score of 23, noting that this indicates enough concern to warrant a more in-depth screening or assessment. When he protested, she showed him the means chart for his age group, noting that "clinical samples" are the individuals who needed further intervention. She assured him that she would work with him and that the school would not try to punish him. He expressed anger and fear. The social worker calmly and firmly explained the next steps and gave him some choices so that he could feel empowered. Because of the reference to marijuana, the worker noted that the follow-up should include a more extensive substance abuse history and assessment. This worker was familiar with several students in the school who were young people in 12-Step recovery. She was aware that students at this age talk more freely with peers than with authorities. Thus, she offered that Phil could talk to someone who had been "in the same boat" if he would like to. The social worker had already done "her homework" and had a list of referrals to be considered for Phil to participate in a substance abuse assessment. She also made another appointment with him to explore social supports and see if and who he would be willing to have involved, such as family or friends.

Key Points to Remember

- This chapter aims to provide awareness of the scope and repercussions of adolescent substance abuse, directions for choosing and utilizing a screening tool in school settings, and an example of a screening scenario. Tools including the teacher's behavioral checklist, POSIT, and RAPI are evidence-supported, reliable, simple instruments for gathering information that can help school mental health professionals determine if an adolescent is in need of more intensive substance-related referral and triage. It is important to note, however, that screening tools, no matter how comprehensive, cannot elicit definitive diagnoses and will not be likely to fully capture the nature of an adolescent's relationship to substances. Owing to the fact that adolescents almost always hide their use because of fear, shame, and a desire to maintain the option to use substances, workers must be gentle, creative, and tenacious. The critical data lie in the rapport built between worker and student. In order to do the effective "detective work" of drawing out the facts, building connection with the individual, and putting the pieces together, a worker can utilize motivational interviewing techniques described in other areas of this book (for information, trainings, and publications, see the MI Web site, http://www.motivationalinterview.org).
- It is important to remember that adolescent substance use/abuse can be profoundly injurious mentally, emotionally, socially, and physically. In fact, it can be potentially fatal and should not be minimized as a "passing phase." Workers do best to err on the side of being conservative and, if concerns arise, to consult with and/or refer the student to a substance abuse expert.

Notes

1. The POSIT questionnaire and brief explanation are available at http://www.niaaa.nih.gov/publications/insposit.htm and http://www.niaaa.nih.gov/publications/posit.htm, respectively.
2. Recently, the RAPI authors developed a new version of the scale (18-item) and are testing its psychometric properties.

Effective HIV Prevention in Schools

4

Laura Hopson

Getting Started

Although the overall incidence of AIDS in the United States is declining, there has not been any such improvement in the prevalence among American youth (Centers for Disease Control and Prevention [CDC], 2002). Between 2000 and 2003, the number of HIV/AIDS cases increased among 13- to 14-year-olds and among those between the ages of 15 and 24. There are more heterosexual adolescents infected with HIV/AIDS now than in 2000. Of those males infected with HIV/AIDS over the age of 13, the majority (62%) were men who have sex with men. The majority of females over the age of 13 living with HIV/AIDS were infected through heterosexual contact (CDC, 2003a).

American youth are more likely to have intercourse by age 15 than youth in other Western industrialized countries and are more likely to have multiple, short relationships, which puts them at greater risk (Alan Guttmacher Institute, 2002). In a national survey, over 46% of high school students reported having sexual intercourse, and over 7% had sexual intercourse before age 13. Among those who reported being sexually active, more than 14% reported having sex with four or more partners during their lifetime; only 63% of sexually active students reported using condoms the last time they had intercourse, and over 25% had used drugs or alcohol before their last sexual intercourse (CDC, 2003b). In response to the number of HIV/AIDS cases among American youth, the CDC have made recommendations for preventing HIV/AIDS in this age group. These recommendations include the use of school-based programs because they can reach a great number of youth before they become sexually active. Most adolescents are enrolled in school prior to becoming sexually active and when they are sexually active. Many states now require schools to offer sex education, and most require that schools teach STD/HIV education (Kirby, 2002). The most helpful programs are comprehensive, emphasizing the importance of delaying sexual activity as well as providing information about protection, such as condoms, for sexually active youth (CDC, 2002).

The school setting also presents challenges for providing effective HIV prevention programs. Some schools may not allow condom distribution, for example, which is a component of many effective HIV prevention strategies (Stryker, Samuels, & Smith, 1994). Many schools will only support abstinence-based curricula, especially for younger teens (Lohrmann, Blake, Collins, Windsor, & Parrillo, 2001), which eliminates the majority of research-based HIV prevention programs. Empirical evaluations of abstinence-only curricula have not reliably demonstrated effectiveness in delaying sexual activity (Kirby, 2002). Because of such barriers, it is important that HIV prevention strategies include community intervention and planning, public information campaigns, and policy-level interventions as well as effective school-based programs (CDC, 2003c).

What We Know

Many research-based prevention programs are appropriate for school settings and have demonstrated a range of positive outcomes for adolescents. Programs have been most successful in improving condom use, knowledge about HIV, and communication skills; they have been less successful with reducing overall sexual activity (Collins et al., 2002; Johnson, Carey, Marsh, Levin, & Scott-Sheldon, 2003). Evidence-based prevention programs include a range of components such as instruction, use of video and other media, demonstration of correct condom use, role-plays, and group discussion. The programs described here are defined as evidence-based because they meet one of three criteria: they have been evaluated in experimental design studies that employ random assignment to treatment conditions; they have been evaluated in quasi-experimental designs that use matching; or they are statistically corrected for differences in experimental and comparison groups to compensate for using nonrandom assignment. The evidence-based programs also resulted in statistically significant reductions in sexual risk behaviors. See Table 4.1 for a list of evidence-based programs and their supporting studies.

The outcomes for many of the evidence-based programs included increased condom use (Coyle et al., 1999; Fisher, Fisher, Bryan, & Misovich, 1998; Kirby, Barth, Leland, & Fetro, 1991; Main et al., 1994; Rotheram-Borus, Gwadz, Fernandez & Srinivasan, 1998; St. Lawrence et al., 1995). Other interventions have resulted in less frequent sexual intercourse and fewer sexual partners (Jemmott, Jemmott, & Fong, 1992; Main et al., 1994), as well as delayed initiation of sexual intercourse (Kirby et al., 1991). Because of the need for culturally appropriate HIV prevention, some effective programs have been tailored to meet the needs of students from particular cultural and ethnic backgrounds (Jemmott et al., 1992; Jemmott, Jemmott, Fong, & McCaffree, 1998; Kipke, Boyer, & Hein, 1993; St. Lawrence et al., 1995). Others have been tailored for use with gay and bisexual adolescents (Remafedi, 1994; Rotheram-Borus, Reid, & Rosario, 1994). Rotheram-Borus, Kooperman, Haignere, and Davies (1991) and Rotheram-Borus, Van Rossem, Gwadz, Koopman, and Lee (1997) have also developed an intervention for runaway youth, although the program can be adapted for use with other adolescents as well. Most evidence-based HIV prevention programs share common

Table 4.1 Evidence-Based HIV Prevention Programs

Evidence-Based Interventions:
ARREST Program

Supporting Studies:
Kipke, M. D., et al. (1993). An evaluation of an AIDS risk reduction education and skills training (ARREST) program. *Journal of Adolescent Health, 14*(7), 533–539.

Contact Information:
Michele D. Kipke, Ph.D.
Children's Hospital
P.O. Box 54700
Mailstop #2
Los Angeles, CA 90054–0700

Evidence-Based Interventions:
Be Proud! Be Responsible!

Supporting Studies:
Jemmott, J., et al. (1992). Reductions in HIV risk associated sexual behaviors among black male adolescents: Effects of an AIDS prevention program. *American Journal of Public Health, 82*(3), 372–377.

Contact Information:
John B. Jemmott III, Ph.D.
jjemmott@asc.upenn.edu
Treatment manual available from www.selectmedia.org

Evidence-Based Interventions:
Becoming a Responsible Teen

Supporting Studies:
St. Lawrence, J., et al. (1995). A cognitive-behavioral intervention to reduce African-American adolescents' risk for HIV infection. *Journal of Consulting and Clinical Psychology, 63*(2), 221–237.

Contact Information:
Janet S. St. Lawrence, Ph.D.
nzs4@cdc.gov
Treatment manual available from www.etr.org

Evidence-Based Interventions:
Cognitive and Behavioral Adaptations to HIV/AIDS among Gay and Bisexual Adolescents

Supporting Studies:
Remafedi, G., (1994). Cognitive and behavioral adaptations to HIV/AIDS among gay and bisexual adolescents. *Journal of Adolescent Health, 15,* 142–148.

(continued)

Table 4.1 (Continued)

Contact Information:
  Gary Remafedi, MD
  Box 721 UMHC
  420 Delaware St. SE
  Minneapolis, MN 55455–0392

Evidence-Based Interventions:
  Factors Mediating Changes in Sexual HIV Risk Behaviors among Gay and
  Bisexual Male Adolescents

Supporting Studies:
  Rotheram-Borus, M. J., et al. (1994). Factors mediating changes in sexual HIV risk
  behaviors among gay and bisexual male adolescents. American Journal of Public
  Health, 84(12), 1938–1946.

Contact Information:
  Mary Jane Rotheram-Borus, Ph.D.
  rotheram@ucla.edu

Evidence-Based Interventions:
  Focus on Kids

Supporting Studies:
  Stanton, B., et al. (1996). A randomized, controlled effectiveness trial of an
  AIDS prevention program for low-income African-American youths. Archives
  of Pediatric and Adolescent Medicine, 151(4), 398–406.

Contact Information:
  Bonita Stanton, MD
  bstanton@umabnet.ab.umd
  Educational treatment manual available from www.etr.org

Evidence-Based Interventions:
  Get Real About AIDS

Supporting Studies:
  Main, D., et al. (1994). Preventing HIV infection among adolescents: Evaluation
  of a school-based education program. Preventive Medicine, 23(4), 409–417.

Contact Information:
  Deborah S. Main, Ph.D.
  debbi.main@uchsc.edu
  Treatment manual available from AGC Educational Media at agcmedia@
  starnetinc.com

Evidence-Based Interventions:
  Information-Motivation-Behavioral Skills Model–Based HIV Prevention
  Curriculum

(continued)

Table 4.1 *(Continued)*

Supporting Studies:
Fisher, J. D., et al. (1998). Information- motivation-behavioral skills model- based HIV risk behavior change intervention for inner city youth. *Health Psychology, 21*(2), 177–186.

Contact Information:
Jeffrey Fisher, Ph.D.
jeffrey.fisher@uconn.edu
Videos and treatment manual available from www.films.org

Evidence-Based Interventions:
Making a Difference

Supporting Studies:
Jemmott, J., et al. (1998). Abstinence and safer sex HIV risk reduction interventions for African American adolescents. Journal of the American Medical Association, 279(19), 1529–1536.

Contact Information:
John B. Jemmott III, Ph.D.
jjemmott@asc.upenn.edu
Treatment manual available from www.selectmedia.org

Evidence-Based Interventions:
Making Proud Choices

Supporting Studies:
Jemmott, J., et al. (1998). Abstinence and safer sex HIV risk reduction interventions for African American adolescents. *Journal of the American Medical Association, 279*(19), 1529–1536.

Contact Information:
John B. Jemmott III, Ph.D.
jjemmott@asc.upenn.edu
Treatment manual available from www.selectmedia.org

Evidence-Based Interventions:
Reducing the Risk

Supporting Studies:
Kirby, D., et al. (1991). Reducing the risk: Impact of a new curriculum on sexual risk-taking. *Family Planning Perspectives, 23*(6), 253–263.

Contact Information:
Nancy Shanfeld, Ph.D.
ETR Associates
Treatment manual available from www.etr.org

(continued)

Table 4.1 *(Continued)*

Evidence-Based Interventions:
Safer Choices

Supporting Studies:
Coyle, K., et al. (1999). Short term impact of Safer-Choices: A multi-component, school-based HIV, other STD, and pregnancy prevention program. *Journal of School Health, 69*(5), 181–188.

Contact Information:
Karin Coyle, Ph.D.
(831) 438–4060, ext. 140
Treatment manual available from www.etr.org

Evidence-Based Interventions:
Self Center

Supporting Studies:
Zabin, L. S., et al. (1988). The Baltimore Pregnancy Prevention Program for urban teenagers: 1. How did it work? *Family Planning Perspectives, 20,* 182–187.

Contact Information:
Laurie Schwab Zabin, Ph.D.
Johns Hopkins University
Sociometrics, Program Archive on Sexuality, Health & Adolescence
http://www.socio.com

Evidence-Based Interventions:
Street Smart

Supporting Studies:
Rotheram-Borus, M., et al. (1997). *Street Smart.*

Contact Information:
Mary Jane Rotheram-Borus, Ph.D.
rotheram@ucla.edu
Intervention manual available from http://chipts.ucla.edu/interventions/manuals/intervstreetsmart.html

Evidence-Based Interventions:
3 Week and 7 Week HIV Interventions

Supporting Studies:
Rotheram-Borus, M., et al. (1998). Timing of HIV interventions on reductions in sexual risk among adolescents. *American Journal of Community Psychology, 26,* 73–96.

Contact Information:
Mary Jane Rotheram- Borus, Ph.D.
rotheram@ucla.edu

core components. Box 4.1 displays a list of characteristics identified by Kirby (1999) that are found in effective programs.

Fisher et al. (1998) found that students participating in a 5-day classroom curriculum had increased knowledge about HIV, were more likely to use

Box 4.1. Common Core Components of Most Evidence-Based HIV Prevention Programs

According to Kirby (1999), most evidence-based programs have the following characteristics:

1. A focus on reducing one or more sexual risk behaviors
2. A foundation in theoretical approaches that are effective in influencing the health behaviors that are the focus of the intervention
3. A clear message and consistent reinforcing of the health behaviors
4. Clear, accurate information about the risks associated with sexual behaviors and how to avoid unprotected sexual intercourse
5. A component that addresses peer pressure to engage in sexual behaviors
6. Use of modeling and opportunities for participants to practice communication, negotiation, and refusal skills
7. Diverse teaching methods that involve participants and allow them to personalize the curriculum
8. Behavioral goal setting and teaching methods that are appropriate to the age, sexual experience, and culture of participants
9. Adequate duration to allow participants time to complete activities
10. Selection of people who believe in the program to be trained and lead the curriculum

From "Reflections on two decades of research on teen sexual behavior and pregnancy," by D. Kirby, 1999. *Journal of School Health, 69*(3), 89–94.

condoms, and had more positive attitudes about HIV prevention behaviors. In the curriculum, students learn factual information about HIV, watch videos and participate in activities designed to increase motivation for reducing HIV risk behaviors, and learn skills for reducing risk behaviors. The following section provides a case example of a school that implements Fisher et al.'s (1998) program and summarizes the curriculum activities.

Tools and Practice Examples

Case Example: Newton High School

Ms. Jones, the principal at Newton High School, is concerned about the large number of pregnant and parenting teens at Newton. In order to better understand the problem, Ms. Jones meets with the school social worker, nurse, and counselors. The social worker and nurse report that several students have expressed concerns related to sexually transmitted diseases and pregnancy. They feel that students need more education about reducing risk because students often ask about safe sex practices and contraception. The counselors agree that students lack adequate knowledge about sexual risks and effective protection. Ms. Jones also learns that the community surrounding Newton has higher rates of sexually transmitted diseases than other communities in the district, and HIV rates among young adults in her community are higher than average.

Ms. Jones decides that she needs an effective HIV prevention program at Newton to protect her students. Because many of her students are already sexually active, Ms. Jones chooses Fisher et al.'s (1998) classroom-based curriculum, which helps students learn skills to abstain from sexual activity as well as skills for using contraception. Because the curriculum uses videotapes to provide much of the information on HIV prevention information and skills, Ms. Jones also felt that it would be relatively easy for her teachers to implement. Ms. Quincy is one of several Newton High School teachers who volunteer to provide the curriculum to their classes. Ms. Quincy teaches an English class in which she meets with the same group of 10th graders every day. During this week, 40 minutes of class time will be devoted to the Information-Motivation-Behavioral Skills Curriculum. The following overview of sessions is based on the teacher's manual for the curriculum available from www.films.com (Misovich et al., 2000).

Information-Motivation-Behavioral Skills
HIV Prevention Program

Day 1

The Information-Motivation-Behavioral Skills Curriculum consists of five 40-minute sessions that are provided to students on consecutive class days. During the first session, students learn facts about HIV transmission and prevention. The session also aims to correct common misperceptions about HIV. Students watch the video "Knowing the Facts: Preventing Infection" and participate in classroom activities. After the video, students discuss the following three ways that HIV can be transmitted from one person to another: unprotected sexual intercourse, sharing needles, and transmission from mother to baby during pregnancy, birth, or breastfeeding. The group also discusses abstinence from sexual intercourse as an HIV prevention behavior and correct condom use as a behavior that greatly reduces risk for transmission of HIV.

In one of the activities for this session, students are given flashcards with questions about HIV risk behaviors, and they answer the questions for the group. One flashcard, for example, lists several behaviors, and students are asked to say whether the behavior is high risk, low risk, or no risk for HIV transmission. These behaviors include French kissing, oral sex, vaginal or anal intercourse using a condom correctly and without a condom, and sharing needles.

Group Discussion and Flashcard Activity With Ms. Quincy's Class After Ms. Quincy shows her students the video "Knowing the Facts: Preventing Infection," she asks students to discuss the three ways that HIV can be transmitted from one person to another. The students were able to talk about each of the three ways: unprotected sexual intercourse, sharing needles, and from mother to baby. In response to another of Ms. Quincy's questions about ways to prevent transmission of HIV, the students say that using condoms will prevent HIV. Ms. Quincy asks the students if condoms are 100% effective at preventing transmission, and the students respond that, if a condom breaks or is not used properly, it may not be effective.

Ms. Quincy distributes flashcards to the students for the activity. Each flashcard displays a question, and the students are asked to read the question out loud and answer it. She explains that some of the flashcards ask about sexual behaviors that might be a little difficult to talk about but that the group can contribute by answering the questions. Ms. Quincy asks one of her students, Jessica, to begin. Jessica stands and reads the question on her card, "How can you tell if a person is infected with HIV?" Jessica says that she does not think that you can tell if a person has HIV by their appearance. Ms. Quincy tells Jessica that she is correct because most people with HIV do not have symptoms that are visible to others.

The next student, Jason, reads the question on his card, "What are high risk, low risk, and no risk behaviors for transmitting HIV?" Jason reads the first behavior on the flashcard, "French kissing," and says that this behavior presents no risk because HIV cannot be passed from one person to another through saliva. Jason reads another behavior on the flashcard "Vaginal or anal intercourse always using a condom properly," and says that he thinks this behavior is no risk but he is not sure. Ms. Quincy asks the class to discuss this, and several students agree with Jason that the behavior is no risk. Other students say that the behavior presents some risk because a condom could break even if it is used properly. Ms. Quincy says that it is true that the condom can break, so the behavior would be classified as low risk instead of no risk. The group continues this activity until all of the flashcard questions have been discussed and answered.

Day 2

The second class in the curriculum aims to increase students' motivation to practice HIV prevention behaviors. The session includes showing the video "Just Like Me: Talking About AIDS," in which young people infected with HIV ask that students change their attitudes about HIV risk so they can prevent becoming infected as well. Following the video, teachers facilitate a discussion about how the attitudes and norms that led to the infection of the people in the video are common among many teens. This session also includes a group discussion about abstaining from sexual activity that includes reasons people may want to wait until they are older to have sexual intercourse, why it might be difficult to wait, and strategies for making it less difficult to wait. Following this discussion, the teacher facilitates another discussion about using condoms.

Day 2 Curriculum With Ms. Quincy's Class   After the class watches the video, Ms. Quincy asks the students, "What were some of the reasons that people in the video mentioned that made them think they could not be infected by the other person?" One of the students, Kelly, responds, "One of the assumptions was that if you are in a committed relationship with one person for a long time, you can't get HIV." Another student says, "They also thought that because they were young they couldn't get HIV." Ms. Quincy asks, "How common are these assumptions among people you know?" The students agree that many of their peers would think that they are safe if they are having sex with young people because they do not believe that young people are going to have HIV. Ms. Quincy asks the students to also discuss how the people in the video said others can avoid getting HIV. The students respond that using condoms correctly can reduce their risk and abstaining from sex can prevent HIV altogether.

Day 3

The third session aims to further motivate participants with a third video, "Stakes are High: Asserting Yourself Part I," which features real high school students overcoming obstacles to HIV prevention by assertively negotiating abstinence or using contraception. In the video, students also support each other for using HIV prevention strategies. Students in the group participate in classroom activities and group discussion that encourage peer support of HIV prevention behaviors. The session also includes a discussion about how to obtain and carry condoms.

Day 3 Group Discussion With Ms. Quincy's Class   The discussion following the video begins with Ms. Quincy's asking the class about two of the high school students in the video, Afiya and Tyrone. Afiya has decided that she does not want to have sex until she is married. The class discusses the strategies that Afiya uses to make it less difficult for her to abstain from sexual activity. One student says that a strategy Afiya uses is to suggest that the couple leave the apartment where they would be alone and more likely to have sex. Another student says that Afiya was also direct and firm with Tyrone in telling him that she would not have sex until she was married. Ms. Quincy asks the class to discuss another couple in the video who decided that they might want to have sex but had no condoms. The students discussed how friends in the video were able to support the couple by strongly advising them to use condoms and going with them when they went to buy condoms.

In order to encourage the students to think about the logistics of obtaining condoms, Ms. Quincy asks them to discuss a scene in the video in which students purchase condoms. She asks students about convenient places where they might go to get condoms. One of the students mentions that the drug store two blocks from the school would probably have condoms. Another student says that the school nurse might also have condoms that she would give to students. Ms. Quincy agrees that those are both places that are likely to have condoms.

Day 4

The fourth session aims to help students develop behavioral skills for abstinence and condom use. The session includes a fourth video, "Stakes Are High: Asserting Yourself Part 2," which shows adolescents demonstrating HIV prevention behaviors, such as abstaining from sex, discussing condoms, and using condoms. Students then practice these behaviors themselves. The teacher demonstrates correctly placing a condom over fingers or a model of a penis, and students then practice doing the same. The teacher gives students scripts printed on large cards from which they can practice negotiating abstinence from sex or condom use with a partner.

Practicing Negotiation Skills With Ms. Quincy's Class   Ms. Quincy distributes large cards, each of which displays an important step in practicing safer sex through condom use. The cards include statements such as "Decision to Have Intercourse," "Discuss Methods of Birth Control," "Decide to Use Condoms," "Get Condoms," "Take Condom Out of Package," and "Unroll Condom on Erect Penis." Ms. Quincy asks the students to hold their cards and form a line so that their cards are displayed in the correct order of steps for practicing safer sex. After about 15 minutes, the students have placed themselves in the correct order. Ms. Quincy then asks them to read aloud and discuss each step.

Jessica is the first in the row of students and she reads her card, "Decision to Have Intercourse." Ms. Quincy asks the students to talk about how they would make this decision. Jessica begins by saying that the couple should consider whether they both really want to have intercourse or whether one partner is putting pressure on the other. Another student, David, adds that this would be the time for the couple to think about the social and physical consequences of intercourse. Ms. Quincy asks David to give an example of a social and a physical consequence. David says that having sex might take their relationship to a more serious level and make it more painful if the couple ended the relationship. He adds that the physical consequences could be pregnancy or getting HIV. Ms. Quincy continues to facilitate the discussion by asking each student to read their card and discuss how they would complete the step.

Day 5

The final session is a review of communication strategies. The students then form small groups and generate their own responses to common scenarios that increase risk for HIV. The group provides feedback on the students' responses according to the communication skills discussed during previous sessions. Students' responses are critiqued and modified by their peers and the teacher to become more effective for preventing HIV risk behavior. Students then have the opportunity to practice using the modified responses.

Practicing Communication in Ms. Quincy's Class   In one of the small groups, a female student, Jessica, is practicing a response to peer pressure from her boyfriend to have sexual intercourse. A male student, David, is playing the role of the boyfriend. David says to Jessica, "I don't understand why you don't want to have sex with me. You must not care about me, or maybe you're more interested in someone else." Jessica responds by saying, "That's not true. I just don't want to have sex until I'm out of high school at least." David continues to press Jessica by saying that he does not understand and feels hurt. Jessica offers the same response each time.

Ms. Quincy asks the other students in the group to help Jessica by using some of the communication skills they have learned. One of the students asks Jessica if she could tell David that she does care about David and wants to be with him but that there are other things they can do together that will strengthen their relationship. Another student suggests that Jessica be firmer in telling her boyfriend that she will not have sex. Jessica practices this response: "David, I care about you very much. Even though I won't have sex, there are a lot of things I want to do with you and I want our relationship to be strong. What else can we do together?" In order to reinforce this behavior, the group tells Jessica that she handled the situation well by communicating to David firmly that she would not have sex but that the relationship was important to her.

A description of the sessions described above is provided in Fisher et al.'s (1998) article describing the study evaluating the curriculum. A treatment manual for sessions 1 through 4 and the videos used in each session are available from www.films.org

Resources

Advocates for Youth: www.advocatesforyouth.org

The Centers for Disease Control and Prevention Division of Sexually Transmitted Diseases: http://www.cdc.gov/std/

The Centers for Disease Control and Prevention Division of HIV/AIDS Prevention: http://www.cdc.gov/hiv/dhap.htm

The Centers for Disease Control and Prevention's Compendium of HIV Prevention Interventions with Evidence of Effectiveness: http://www.cdc.gov/hiv/pubs/ HIVcompendium/hivcompendium.htm

The Center for HIV Identification, Prevention, and Treatment Services (CHIPTS): http://chipts.ucla.edu/about/index.html

Sociometrics HIV/AIDS Prevention Program Archive (HAPPA): http://www.socio. com/pasha/haprogms.htm

Southwestern University's HIV Prevention Toolbox: http://www3.utsouthwestern. edu/preventiontoolbox/interven.htm

Key Points to Remember

Some of the key points discussed in this chapter were:

- The prevalence of HIV/AIDS among adolescents and young adults indicates a great need to reduce sexual risk behaviors among American youth.

- A number of evidence-based HIV prevention programs are appropriate for use in schools, and school-based curricula have the potential to reach many teens before they become sexually active as well as those who are already sexually active.

- Most of the effective HIV prevention curricula include educational and skill-building components.

- Fisher et al.'s (1998) Information-Motivation-Behavioral Skills curriculum is one approach that has resulted in increased condom use and more positive attitudes about HIV prevention behaviors when administered to teens in a school setting.

There is a great need for interventions that reduce risk for HIV/AIDS among youth. Fortunately, many effective and promising programs have already been developed. The challenge for the future will be to work with schools and other organizations to help them implement these evidence-based programs. Because the curricula include information about condom use as well as abstinence from sexual intercourse, school staff may face opposition when trying to implement these programs, and successful implementation may require advocating for changes in state and local school policies.

5 | Effective STD Prevention

Laura Hopson

Getting Started

According to the Youth Risk Behavior Surveillance conducted by the Centers for Disease Control and Prevention (CDC), almost half of American high school students have had sex in their lifetime, and over one third reported being currently sexually active. Of these students, only 63% reported using condoms the last time they had intercourse (CDC, 2003b). The high rates of sexual activity and failure to use condoms in many cases helps explain the large number of American adolescents infected with sexually transmitted diseases (STDs).

Although rates of gonorrhea infection have generally declined among American youth, women between the ages of 15 and 19 represent the largest proportion of women diagnosed with gonorrhea at a rate of about 635 cases per every 100,000 women in this age group. Infection rates for gonorrhea among male adolescents are about 466 per every 100,000 males between the ages of 15 and 19. *Chlamydia* infection is widespread and especially problematic among economically disadvantaged women. The Adolescent Women Reproductive Health Monitoring Project estimates that more than 11% of adolescent women are infected with *Chlamydia* (CDC, 2003a). Adolescent girls may be at higher risk than adult women for becoming infected with STDs because of their immature cervix. They are also more likely to have multiple partners within a short period and older partners who may have multiple partners themselves.

STD prevention programs for adolescents face many challenges because adolescents often do not perceive themselves to be at risk. They may hold negative beliefs about condom use and have few skills to negotiate safer sex practices with a partner. Programs may face additional barriers because those that discuss condom use are controversial in many communities. As with HIV prevention strategies, effective STD prevention may require addressing political barriers and misinformation, including the idea that sex education results in increased sexual activity among teens (CDC, 2003a).

What We Know

A summary of interventions that effectively reduce HIV risk behaviors among adolescents is provided in Chapter 4. These programs are also effective in preventing STDs. See Table 4.1 for a list of evidence-based programs that are appropriate for use in a school setting.

One of these effective programs is Street Smart, a program developed by Rotheram-Borus, Van Rossem, Gwadz, Koopman, and Lee (1997) for use with runaway youth. The treatment manual specifies that this curriculum may be easily adapted for use with other adolescents as well. In adapting the curriculum, however, it is important to maintain the critical, core components of the intervention displayed in Box 5.1 (Southwestern, n.d.). Without including all of these core components, the intervention may lose some of its effectiveness. The curriculum consists of eight 2-hour group sessions, one individual session, and a session in which the group visits a community agency. Each session of the Street Smart curriculum includes the key techniques displayed in Box 5.2.

In a study evaluating the effects of Street Smart with runaway youth, teens who received the intervention reduced the number of unprotected sexual acts and reduced their substance use when compared with teens who did not receive the intervention. The following description of sessions is based on information

Box 5.1. Core Elements of the Street Smart Program

Core elements are components that must be included in the program as indicated in the manual in order for the program to maintain its effectiveness. For Street Smart, these elements are as follows:

- Opportunities to practice controlling and expressing emotions and cognitive awareness
- Teaching HIV/AIDS risks and allowing participants opportunities to apply the ideas to their own lives
- Identifying personal triggers for HIV risk behaviors
- Using peer support and skills-building in small groups
- Building skills in problem solving, assertiveness, and skills for reducing HIV/AIDS risk behaviors

Source: From *HIV prevention toolbox: Street smart,* by Southwestern, The University of Texas Southwestern Medical Center at Dallas, n.d. Retrieved December 21, 2004 from http://www3.utsouthwestern.edu/preventiontoolbox/interven/streetsmart.htm

Box 5.2. Key Components of Every Street Smart Session

1. A stack of tokens, which are 1" × 1" pieces of colored paper, are given to each participant. When participants hear or see another group member doing something that they like, they give that group member a token.

2. A feeling thermometer is a scale that ranges from 0 to 100, with 100 representing the most discomfort and 0 representing a complete absence of discomfort. Facilitators use the thermometer to help participants recognize, assess, and discuss their feelings.

3. Role-playing in each session gives participants the opportunity to practice new behaviors and act out situations in a supportive environment. Role-plays in Street Smart session consist of two actors playing out a scene, a coach assigned to each actor to provide suggestions, one director who determines who plays each part, and other participants assigned to observe interactions, such as eye contact and body language, during the role-play.

4. The sessions are videotaped so that students can observe themselves interacting in the role-play situations.

5. Participants use the SMART model to apply the following problem-solving steps:
   a. State the problem
   b. Make a goal
   c. Actions—list the possible actions that could be taken
   d. Reach a decision about which action to use
   e. Try doing the action and review it

6. A large flipchart on a stand is used to save written material and goals set by participants so that they can be reviewed later.

7. The curriculum provides choices in the curriculum so that facilitators have different options they can use with their participants for each session.

Source: From Street Smart, by M. Rotheram-Borus, R. Van Rossem, M. Gwadz, C. Koopman, & M. Lee, 1997. Retrieved December 18, 2004 from http://chipts.ucla.edu/interventions/manuals/intervstreetsmart.html

provided in the treatment manual for Street Smart, which can be downloaded from the following Web site: http://chipts.ucla.edu (Rotheram-Borus et al., 1997).

Tools and Practice Examples

Case Example: Jenson High School

Ms. Davis is a social worker at Jenson High School, an alternative school for students who have experienced behavioral or academic difficulties that made it difficult for them to thrive at a traditional high school. Students often come to Ms. Davis to ask her questions about sexual health, and a number of students at Jenson are pregnant or parenting teens. Because Ms. Davis suspects that many of the students engage in a number of risk behaviors, such as unprotected sexual activity and drug use, she administers an anonymous survey to the student body. The results of the survey suggest that 60% of the students at Jenson are sexually active, and 40% use alcohol or drugs on a regular basis. Other results that concern Ms. Davis include a large number of sexually active students who indicated that they do not use condoms when they have sex or that they consume alcohol or drugs prior to having sex.

Ms. Davis takes the results to the principal and asks permission to implement a program designed to reduce sexual risk taking. The principal agrees that Ms. Davis should work to find a program that will reduce risks for students at Jenson. Ms. Davis decides on the Street Smart program because it provides information about STDs and HIV, condom use, and the risks of combining alcohol or drug use with sexual activity. With the approval of the principal, Ms. Davis sends parents of the students permission letters that describe the curriculum. Ms. Davis gives students who have parental permission to participate the opportunity to join the group activity, which will take place after school.

Street Smart

Session 1: Getting the Language of HIV and STDs

The first day of Street Smart is dedicated to learning facts about HIV and STDs as well as learning about situations that present great risks for transmission of HIV and STDs. This session begins with introductions and the "Be Smart about HIV/AIDS and STDs" game in which participants form teams and answer questions about HIV/AIDS and STDs. Following the game, participants engage in role-playing and discuss situations in which they would feel high, moderate, low, and no discomfort, using the feeling thermometer for illustration. See Box 5.2 for a description of the feeling thermometer. Another activity included in this session involves giving students nametags, some of which display a small star or square indicating that the person is HIV positive or has an STD. This activity helps students to see how easily and quickly HIV and STDs can be spread to uninfected people. The session concludes with a discussion about participants' strengths and resources that can help them achieve their goals.

Nametag Activity With Jenson High School Students   Ms. Davis provides nametags to all of the participants. Two of the nametags have a small square in the corner, and two others have a small star. The students put on the nametags, and Ms. Davis asks them to pretend they are at a party, mingling with the other group members. Ms. Davis asks the students to identify at least two situations that would be triggers for risky sexual behavior and discuss them with others. She also tells them to identify someone as a potential romantic partner.

After a few minutes of mingling, Ms. Davis asks the students to talk about the triggers for engaging in risky behavior. She then explains that two people in the group have a small star on their nametag and that these two group members represent people who are HIV positive. Two other people, she explains, have small squares on their nametags, representing people who have an STD. After a few minutes, the group members have discovered which group members are wearing the nametags in question. Ms. Davis explains that, if anyone in the group had engaged in risky sexual behavior with those people, they may have contracted STD or HIV and passed it on to others. Ms. Davis encourages group members to discuss the exercise.

Session 2: Personalized Risk

In this session, participants begin by discussing how old they were when they had their first serious relationship. They role-play a situation in which they define a risk behavior and the triggers associated with the behavior. For example, two students enact a script in which a girl tells her friend that she had sex without using protection, and the friend questions her behavior. The role-play is followed by questions about what the girl's triggers were for unsafe sex and what skills might have helped her avoid unsafe sex. Students divide into two groups and create a list of possible triggers for having unsafe sex, and participants write down a personal trigger that puts them at risk for unsafe sex. In another role-play, participants practice setting their own limits. The facilitator also encourages group members to express appreciation for the contributions of other members.

Session 3: How to Use Condoms

The session begins with a discussion about the best color for a box of condoms. Each participant receives several condoms to handle in order to reduce discomfort with condoms. In order to encourage the students, the facilitator may say, "Open up the condoms and do whatever you want with them—stretch them, chew on them, whatever." The group is then asked to try to figure out the correct steps in putting on a male condom. Participants practice putting male condoms on a penis model and female condoms in the female model. The facilitator can ask the participants to use the feeling thermometer to monitor any feelings of discomfort during these activities.

Session 4: Drugs and Alcohol

This session begins with a discussion about any successes students have had in practicing behavior related to previous sessions. Through a role-playing activity, participants explore the relationship between drug and alcohol use and sexual risk behavior. The students also make a list of the advantages and disadvantages of substance use. Another role-play is used to help participants understand how substance use affects their ability to practice safer sex. The facilitator presents information about the effect of substance use on the brain and asks participants to identify triggers that put them at risk for using substances, along with ways to deal with those triggers. A third role-play helps students deal with risky situations.

Discussing Beliefs About Alcohol and Drug Use With Jenson High School Students   Ms. Davis distributes cards to each of the group members. Each card displays a substance use belief, such as "Using is the only way to increase my creativity and productivity." She then tells the students to imagine that someone has told them that they believe the statement printed on the card and asks them to argue against the belief. In order to model this activity, Ms. Davis asks one of the students to pick a card and hand it to her. She reads the card out loud, "The only way to deal with my anger is by using." In response to the statement, Ms. Davis adds, "Actually, using does not help you deal with the anger at all. It's just a way to keep you from dealing with the thing that's really making you angry." Ms. Davis asks one of the students, Jamie, to practice the activity. Jamie reads her card, "My life won't get better, even if I stop using." Jamie then states her response, "Drug use can cause so many problems—conflicts with your parents, problems with money, failing in school. At least if you weren't using drugs you wouldn't have those problems to deal with." Ms. Davis tells Jamie that she did a wonderful job answering the question and proceeds to ask the next student to read his card and think of a response.

Session 5: Recognizing and Coping With Feelings

Participants begin this session by describing something about themselves that makes them proud. Using the feeling thermometer, participants rate sexually risky situations according to the amount of discomfort they cause. The facilitator may ask students to think of a situation that put them at risk for acquiring an STD and caused a great deal of discomfort, a behavior that they would rate close to 100 on the feeling thermometer. The group thinks about the emotions they feel and any physical stress responses they experience when confronted with the uncomfortable situation, as well as identifying what might have triggered it.

A role-playing activity is used to help participants understand how to cope with risky situations, and a second role-play helps them learn effective problem definition as a strategy for learning to focus on manageable problems. The role-playing continues in this session with a situation in which participants have to get tested for HIV.

Session 6: Negotiating Effectively

Participants begin by reviewing any successes they have had relevant to the previous session. This session includes an opportunity for each group member to consider his or her own sexual values. In order to learn how to deal with peer pressure to engage in substance abuse and risky sexual behavior, participants practice using interpersonal problem-solving skills. They also participate in a role-play in which they have to ask potential sexual partners questions to determine whether they are at risk for having HIV or STDs. The facilitator asks students to generate a list of questions that would be helpful in this situation and ensures that questions such as "Do you usually use a condom?" "Do you shoot drugs?" and "Have you had a lot of sex partners?" are included in the list.

Session 7: Self-Talk

The facilitator begins this session by asking participants to tell the group things that they say to themselves to make them feel good. The facilitator explains that we have thoughts that help us practice healthier behaviors and other thoughts that are barriers to practicing those behaviors. Through participating in a game, group members learn to distinguish between harmful and helpful thoughts related to sexual risk behavior. Group members are given the opportunity to practice moving from harmful thoughts to helpful thoughts through a role-play. The facilitator helps by giving several examples of self-talk statements.

Practicing Self-Talk With Jenson High School Students   Ms. Davis explains to the group that self-talk is something we do all the time, but we do not always realize it. She goes on to say that we can make self-talk helpful for reducing our chances of engaging in risky behavior. In explaining how to use self-talk, Ms. Davis breaks it down into parts. First, she says, you make a plan to confront a situation. Then you act on the situation. If you feel that you are getting overwhelmed, use self-talk to help yourself cope. Finally, you evaluate the situation and how you handled it. Ms. Davis distributes a handout that provides examples of self-talk for each part of the process. For the planning step, examples of self-talk include "This is going to be tough, but I can handle it" and "I'll take a few deep breaths beforehand." For acting on the situation, an example of self-talk would be "Don't let him rattle me" and "I have a right to my point of view." When experiencing feeling overwhelmed, helpful self-talk includes statements such as "He wants me to get angry" and "There's no shame in leaving and coming back later." Ms. Davis asks the class if there are statements they would like to add to the list of self-talk suggestions.

Session 8: Safer Sex

In this session, the participants learn why people sometimes take sexual risks even though they know the behavior is risky. Using the feeling thermometer, participants can assess their own level of discomfort in discussing safer sex. They learn about the kinds of rationalizations that increase risk for unsafe sex and how to deal with those rationalizations. Included in this part of the curriculum is a goal-setting activity to help group members define what they want for themselves. Students make a list of their goals and rate the goals on a scale from 1 to 10, with 1 meaning that the goal is not very important and 10 meaning that the goal is very important. The facilitator personalizes the curriculum by asking group members why they and their friends might engage in risky behaviors. Students can use their creativity in an activity that involves creating a music video, commercial, or other media to create a message promoting safer sex. Since this is the final interactive group session, the participants discuss the conclusions of the group.

Session 9: Personal Counseling

In the personal counseling session, the facilitator assesses whether the participants are sexually active and asks them to identify priorities and goals related to safer sex. The session is also used to help the teens identify triggers that might prevent them from practicing safer sex behaviors and develop a plan for coping with these triggers. The students are then given the opportunity to ask any questions about HIV/AIDS, STDs, testing, community resources, and anything else that they would like to know.

Session 10: Looking Over a Community Resource

For this session, the facilitator takes a group of participants to visit a relevant community resource so that the group can learn more about the services available in their community and can form links with the community agency that provides those services. Before the visit, the facilitator helps the participants develop questions for the staff at the community agency. The staff and consumers at the community agency describe the resources provided by the agency and allow participants to ask questions. To allow more time for discussion, the group may also share a meal with the agency staff and consumers. The facilitator encourages the group to make specific plans to return for another visit and to thank the staff and consumers for the visit.

Resources

Advocates for Youth: www.advocatesforyouth.org
The Centers for Disease Control and Prevention Division of Sexually Transmitted Diseases: http://www.cdc.gov/std/
The Centers for Disease Control and Prevention Division of HIV/AIDS Prevention: http://www.cdc.gov/hiv/dhap.htm

The Centers for Disease Control and Prevention's compendium of HIV prevention interventions with evidence of effectiveness: http:// www.cdc.gov/hiv/pubs/ HIVcompendium/hivcompendium.htm
The Center for HIV Identification, Prevention, and Treatment Services (CHIPTS): http://chipts.ucla.edu/about/index.html
Sociometrics HIV/AIDS Prevention Program Archive (HAPPA): http://www.socio. com/pasha/haprogms.htm
Southwestern University's HIV Prevention Toolbox: http://www3.utsouthwestern. edu/ preventiontoolbox/

Key Points to Remember

The key points discussed in this chapter include:

- Implementation of effective STD prevention programs is greatly needed to reduce the rates of STD infection among American youth.
- One challenge to evidence-based STD prevention is opposition to curricula that discuss safer sax practices, such as condom use.
- The Street Smart program is a 10-session program that has demonstrated reductions in sexual risk taking among runaway youth and can be adapted for use with other adolescents at risk for STDs and HIV.

Many STD and HIV prevention programs have been rigorously evaluated and shown to be effective. In many cases, the authors have also provided user-friendly treatment manuals that are easily accessed. As discussed in Chapter 4, the challenge in implementing these programs will be overcoming some of the barriers to using effective programs that include instruction on safer sex strategies, such as condom use.

Effective Cognitive-Behavioral Interventions for Self-Mutilation

Katherine Shepard
Tamara DeHay
Brooke Hersh

Getting Started

The expression of self-mutilation behaviors (SMBs) in children and adolescents is a frightening and, in some ways, puzzling phenomenon. Often referred to in the literature as *deliberate self-harm, self-mutilation behavior, parasuicidal behavior, partial suicide, antisuicide,* and *wrist-cutting syndrome*, the act of SMB can be defined on the basis of its directness, social acceptability, degree of damage, frequency, and intent (Suyemoto, 1998). Specifically, it has been defined as the direct, deliberate, and repetitive destruction or alteration of body tissue, which results in minor to moderate injury, without conscious suicidal intent (Favazza & Conterio, 1989; Suyemoto, 1998). The behaviors that constitute self-mutilation are diverse and include behaviors such as cutting, burning, scratching, and skin-picking (Simeon & Favazza, 2001). It is distinguished from socially accepted forms of bodily harm such as body piercing or tattooing and from indirect forms such as drinking and driving, and substance abuse.

As mentioned in the definition, it is important to make a clear distinction between the types of SMB discussed here and suicidality. The three characteristics commonly cited as distinguishing between the two are lethality, intent, and repetition. SMB usually results in superficial to moderate injury, with very low lethality and without suicidal intent. It is also highly repetitive, with 30% of cases repeating within 1 year. Many have come to view SMB as a precursor to suicide because about half of all people who commit suicide have a history of self-harm and an estimated 10% of people who engage in an act of self-harm subsequently commit suicide (Gunnell & Frankel, 1994; Harris & Hawton, 1997).

What We Know

Classifications of Self-Mutilation Behavior

The most widely used classification system used for self-mutilation proposes four large categories (Favazza, 1998; Favazza & Rosenthal, 1990; Favazza & Simeon, 1995; Simeon & Favazza, 2001). It is important to note the four-category model is based primarily on work with adult populations. Despite this limitation, the proposed model provides a useful heuristic for school social workers and other mental health professionals who work with youth engaging in SMBs (Simeon & Favazza, 2001).

Stereotypic Self-Mutilation Behavior

Stereotypic SMB is characterized by highly repetitive behaviors such as head-banging, self-hitting, and skin-picking. Stereotypic SMB is frequently observed in populations with mental retardation, autism, and Lesch-Nyhan, Cornelia de Lange, and Prader-Willi syndrome (Simeon & Favazza, 2001).

Major Self-Mutilation Behavior

Major SMB is the most severe of the four categories. This form of SMB is frequently an isolated occurrence that occurs in either a psychotic or an intoxicated state. Behaviors that constitute major SMB are usually life-threatening and include limb amputation, castration, and self-removal of the eyes (Simeon & Favazza, 2001).

Compulsive Self-Mutilation Behavior

The compulsive form of SMB is characterized by behaviors such as hair-pulling, skin-picking, and severe nail-biting. Individuals with this form of SMB frequently report that these behaviors have a ritualized and symbolic component. Compulsive SMB is commonly seen in individuals diagnosed with trichotillomania, obsessive-compulsive disorder, and stereotypic movement disorders (Simeon & Favazza, 2001).

Impulsive Self-Mutilation Behavior

Impulsive SMB is perhaps the broadest of the four categories. The harming behaviors can occur repetitively or occur only once. The SMB frequently has a symbolic element, such as cleansing or punishment. Behaviors associated with this category include burning, superficial and deep cutting, and self-hitting. This form of SMB is frequently observed in individuals diagnosed with personality disorders (mainly borderline), eating disorders, depression, and posttraumatic stress disorder (Simeon & Favazza, 2001).

This review of effective practices with youth with SMB will focus primarily on youth engaging in impulsive SMB.

Prevalence

The prevalence rate of self-mutilation behavior as defined in the earlier section is difficult to assess, and a wide disparity exists between the rates documented in the extant literature. Many patients who have engaged in these behaviors will not report them spontaneously, and because of the lack of severity of the actual physical harm, many cases are never reported even when the individual is explicitly asked. Some research has estimated that SMB occurs in approximately 4% of the general population and in 4.3% to 21% of clinical populations (Suyemoto, 1998).

The age of onset of SMBs is usually in middle to late adolescence and the majority of documented cases have occurred in females (Favazza & Conterio, 1988; Sonneborn & Vanstraelen, 1992; Suyemoto, 1998). There is again much disagreement in the literature regarding the actual prevalence within the adolescent population. For instance, Kahan and Pattison (1984) have reported that the incidence is relatively low at 1.2%, while Favazza, DeRosear, and Conterio (1989) found a prevalence rate of 12% in a general sample of college students.

When adolescents do engage in self-mutilation behavior, it seems that it most often includes skin-cutting and picking at existing wounds. These actions comprise about one third of adolescent self-harm (Guertin, Lloyd-Richardson, Spirito, Donaldson, & Boergers, 2001). They are followed in frequency by acts such as burning and self-hitting (Favazza & Conterio, 1989). A high percentage of people who engage in SMB will repeat the behavior within 1 year, and about 13% of cases are termed "major repeaters," with a lifetime history of five or more episodes (Kreftman & Casey, 1988).

Functions of Self-Mutilation

Most research on impulsive self-mutilation suggests that this behavior is most often used as a coping strategy. Research examining self-mutilation found that it is frequently used by youth who become stressed by the numerous demands that society places upon them as well as by the difficult social transitions that occur during this developmental stage. In a study examining why adolescents cut themselves, Allen (1995) identified three main reasons for cutting:

1. *To manage negative moods.* Most adolescents report feeling intensely angry or distressed immediately preceding the cutting. The subsequent harm serves as a form of self-medication in that the episode releases tension. In addition, adolescents who engage in SMBs report that it ameliorates feelings of depersonalization and alienation from the world. In particular, cutting and burning behaviors appear to make the adolescent feel alive (Allen, 1995).

2. *A response to beliefs or habitual thoughts.* Youth who engage in self-harming behavior also report that it is a way of dealing with a sense of "internal badness" and anger at other individuals. The self-harming behaviors serve as a way to inflict punishment on oneself for having inadequacies as well as to channel aggression toward others back to the self. These explanations for engaging in SMBs are most frequently observed in youths with a history of physical and/or sexual abuse (Allen, 1995).

3. *To manage interactions with others.* To family members and friends of adolescents who engage in SMB, the behaviors are frequently seen as a cry for help or as a method of gaining attention (Allen, 1995). Favazza (1989), however, identified an alternative role that self-mutilation might play in maintaining difficult relationships. In particular, Favazza hypothesizes that "self-mutilators who received nurturance after enduring pain of physical abuse as youngsters may harm themselves as a repetition of their childhood experience because they believe that 'after the suffering there is love and forgiveness.'" Thus, adolescents who engage in self-mutilation may do so as an attempt to obtain love and protection from significant people in their lives.

Adolescents' Experiences During Self-Mutilation

There is a surprising degree of agreement among researchers regarding the phenomenological aspects of self-mutilation behavior. Personal accounts by individuals who engage in SMB often include descriptions of powerful and overwhelming feelings of anger, tension, or anxiety immediately prior to the act. They frequently report experiencing little or no pain during an episode and a sense of relief and invigoration after engaging in cutting (Grossman & Siever, 2001). In this way, the self-mutilation behavior serves to relieve emotional distress and regulate the stress level of the individual. The behavior itself becomes reinforcing to the individual in that it provides a brief reprieve from the intense negative emotions that have triggered it (Favazza, 1999; Herpertz, 1995; Suyemoto, 1998).

Research examining the biological effects of self-mutilation behaviors suggests that such behaviors often trigger the release of neurotransmitters that are associated with decreased stress and increased pleasure. In particular, endogenous opiates appear to serve an important function in SMB (Sandman & Touchette, 2002). Endogenous opiates are released within the body when injury or physical trauma occurs and serve to reduce pain. Thus, one possible function of SMB is to cause the release of endogenous opiates, which results in an "opiate high" where the individual experiences a euphoric-like state. This physiological change is reinforcing because as the individual engages more in self-harming behavior to experience the release of endogenous opiates, his or her system will develop a tolerance for the chemical and require a higher dosage of endogenous opiates to produce the euphoric state. Consequently, the individual will engage in more frequent and severe SMB in order to receive the opiate high (Sandman & Touchette, 2001).

Alternatively, it has been hypothesized that SMB results from insensitivity to pain, which could be due to a chronically elevated level of endogenous opiates. The chronically increased level of these endogenous opiates would result in the individual feeling numb. The pain that they would experience when cutting would serve to counter the numb feeling and decrease sensations of depersonalization and alienation (Sandman & Touchette, 2002). Thus, youth who report cutting to feel alive may have an overabundance of opiates in their systems and cutting may serve to provide a sense of alertness. In sum, research with adult populations suggests that endogenous opiates may play a critical role in creating the positive mental state that individuals experience after cutting.

Factors Associated With Impulsive Self-Mutilation Behavior
Several factors have been identified as being associated with impulsive SMB in adolescents. Among these factors is an overall increased number of risk-taking and reckless behaviors. Additionally, adolescents who engage in SMB frequently present as passive and unable to effectively solve problems. They seem to have overgeneralized memories and marked difficulty in remembering and analyzing specific situations. It may be that their limited access to specific memories renders them less able to use prior experience to find effective means of resolving current problems (Evans, 2000). As mentioned in the previous section, SMB may also be related to dissociation, which results in a feeling of numbness and disconnection from others (van der Kolk & Fisler, 1994). It is important to note that the levels of cognitive and affective disturbance in individuals who engage in SMB are generally higher compared to those in suicide attempters and that this symptomatology may be expressed through multiple self-destructive channels.

Research has identified several risk factors that place youth at greater risk for engaging in SMB. Chapter 7 provides a detailed review of risk factors associated with America's current culture. This chapter focuses exclusively on empirically supported risk factors and interventions for the impulsive form of self-mutilation.

Presence of Other Forms of Psychopathology
As described previously, various forms of psychopathology place youth at greater risk for self-mutilation. Affective and behavioral symptoms such as anxiety, depression, loneliness, conduct problems, antisocial behavior, eating disorders, and anger are often associated with these behaviors. The following description provides a brief description of unique aspects of the relationship between specific diagnoses and self-mutilation.

Depression   Adolescents who are clinically depressed are more likely to engage in self-mutilation. Depressed females who do not receive treatment for depression are at greater risk for using SMB as a means of reducing the symptoms of distress, anxiety, and hopelessness associated with depression (Derouin & Bravender, 2004). In addition to decreasing these symptoms, female adolescents with depression also reported that cutting behaviors elicited care and concern from caregivers when they felt unheard or unnoticed by others.

Eating Disorders   Approximately 60% of adolescent females who report self-mutilation behaviors also report eating disorders (Favazza & Conterio, 1989; Zila & Kiselica, 2001). In adolescents who display both eating disorders and SMB, cutting and other forms of mutilation are utilized as a punishment for binging or failing to follow food restrictions. Yaryura-Tobias, Nezitoglu, and Kaplan's (1995) research also demonstrated that self-mutilation behaviors frequently replace maladaptive eating behaviors in youth who are being treated for anorexia. If, however, the adolescent relapses to an anorectic state, the SMB usually subsides. Consequently, school social workers and other mental health professionals who work with youth with eating disorders must attend to signs that SMB may be occurring.

Borderline Personality Disorder   Borderline personality disorder (BPD) is characterized by intense negative emotions including depression, self-hatred, anger, and hopelessness. Furthermore, individuals with BPD usually lack the coping resources to handle these negative emotions and often resort to SMB or suicide attempts as a form of coping (Ivanoff, Linehan, & Brown, 2001). Thus, it is not surprising that approximately 80% of individuals diagnosed with BPD report having engaged in some form of self-mutilation at least once (Fryer, 1988). Moreover, BPD is the most common diagnosis found in adult populations of self-mutilators (Walsh & Rosen, 1988). Although personality disorders are not diagnosed in children and very rarely diagnosed in adolescents, school social workers and other mental health professionals working with clients who have symptoms consistent with BPD should attend carefully to any signs of suicidal ideation or self-mutilation.

Substance Abuse   An increased rate of substance abuse has been noted in adolescents who engage in SMB. Walsh and Rosen (1988) speculate that this increase is related to the self-mutilating adolescent's overall impulsive pattern of responding. It may also be the case that the substance abuse provides further relief from the adolescent's affective symptoms.

Other Disorders   Bipolar disorder, oppositional defiant disorder, and dysthymia have also been mentioned in the extant literature as disorders associated with SMBs. However, there is a dearth of empirical data on this association; thus, these disorders will not be covered in this chapter.

History of Severe Physical and/or Sexual Abuse

Survivors of either sexual or physical abuse are at greater risk for self-mutilation (Favazza & Conterio, 1989; Pattison & Kahan, 1983; van der Kolk, Perry, & Herman, 1991; Zila & Kiselica, 2001). Physical and sexual abuse by primary caregivers is thought to put children at risk for SMB because the youths must muster all of their own coping resources to handle stress and anxiety without the assistance of their caregiver. Because the level of stressors frequently exceed the level of resources available, the child resorts to the use of maladaptive coping skills, such as cutting, to reduce anxiety (Himber, 1994).

Contagion Factor

Adolescents who are surrounded by peers who engage in self-mutilation practices are at a greater risk for trying these behaviors. Research has demonstrated that youth who are in residential treatment facilities or incarcerated are likely to try cutting or other forms of self-mutilation when exposed to peers who engage in these behaviors (Favazza, 1998; Taiminen, Kallio-Soukainen, Nokso-Koivisto, Kaljonen, & Helenuis, 1998). In addition, there is growing evidence for the contagion factor in "normal" adolescents in the school setting. Self-mutilation is frequently passed among social groups in schools when one child engages in the behavior and reports to peers the relief that he or she experiences as a result of the behavior (Derouin & Bravender, 2004). Thus, school social workers or mental health professionals must carefully monitor students who associate with known self-mutilators.

What We Can Do

Given the high prevalence rate and contagious nature of self-mutilation, it is important that school social workers and other mental health professionals know how to identify and successfully intervene in cases involving cutting or other forms of mutilation. This chapter focuses exclusively on empirically supported cognitive-behavioral and behavioral treatments for SMB. For a review of solution-oriented and strengths-based approaches, see Chapter 7.

Identification and Assessment of SMB

Identifying students who self-mutilate is an extremely difficult task as most youth are highly secretive about these behaviors. Some warning signs that a youth may self-mutilate include wearing long-sleeved clothing in warm weather and wearing many bracelets or wristbands to prevent cuts and scrapes from showing. In addition, these adolescents frequently seek excuses from the school nurse to miss physical education and other outdoor activities that require their skin to be exposed. The school social worker should work closely with school nurses to identify students who demonstrate these warning signs (Derouin & Bravender, 2004).

Once a student has been identified as self-mutilating, it is important that the social worker complete a thorough interview to assess the extent of the mutilating behaviors and the student's current coping strategies. A sample interview will be presented later in this chapter. For additional interviewing strategies and questions, review Chapter 7. In addition to conducting a thorough interview, self-report measures can provide greater insight into the reasons why the student self-mutilates. The Self-Injury Motivation Scale II (SIMS-II; Osuch, Noll, & Putnam, 1999) is a useful tool for assessing the underlying reasons for SMB. This measure identifies six distinct motivations for SMB: (1) affect regulation,

(2) de-isolation, (3) punitive duality, (4) influencing others, (5) magic control, and (6) self-stimulation. Although this scale was developed using adult populations, research has demonstrated that it has adequate psychometric properties for clinical use with adolescents. In addition, SIMS-II has been found to be a useful tool for identifying and quickly assessing a variety of different reasons for the adolescent's SMB. These reasons can be used to provide an initial set of dysfunctional thoughts and beliefs about cutting behavior that can be discussed and challenged in subsequent sessions (Kumar, Pepe, & Steer, 2004).

Predicting Repetition
Because a high percentage of children and adolescents who engage in SMB once will subsequently repeat the behavior (the majority within the first 2 months after the initial act), it is important for school social workers and other mental health professionals to understand the risk factors associated with repetition. Depression and a history of previous SMB significantly increase the risk of repetition. Family functioning is also an important associated factor, and poor parental mental health has been found to be the strongest predictor of repeated self-harm (Chitsabesan, Harrington, Harrington, & Tomenson, 2003). The school social worker must take this into account when meeting with parents about their child's symptoms, and oftentimes it may be helpful to recommend that the parents seek out individual or family counseling.

The Issue of Confidentiality
At some point during the assessment process, it is likely that the school social worker or other mental health professionals will have to inform the adolescent's parents about the behavior. Because of the serious implications that informing the parents can have on the rapport with the adolescent in subsequent sessions, it is important that the school social worker openly discusses the upcoming disclosure with the youth. During this discussion, the social worker should emphasize that parents may be helpful in the recovery process. In addition, the school social worker may want to "brainstorm" ways in which the youth could be involved in the disclosure. In particular, it may be useful for the child to inform his or her parents in the presence of the school social worker during a meeting in the social worker's office (Froeschle & Moyer, 2004).

Promising Interventions
Relatively few empirical studies exist that examine the efficacy of interventions for SMB. Of the few studies that do exist, the majority only explore the efficacy of cognitive-behavioral therapy and behavioral interventions. From this limited body of research, cognitive counseling and behavior modification appear to be effective in adolescent populations. For a review of integrative and strengths-based approaches to treating self-mutilation, see Chapter 7.

Cognitive Counseling

Cognitive therapy educates the client about the relationship between their thoughts, their emotions, and their SMBs. During sessions, the social worker or counselor helps the client identify negative emotions and recognize the relationship between these emotions and thoughts that are associated with self-harming behavior. Then, intervention focuses on helping the client challenge the thoughts that lead to self-mutilation. According to Walsh and Rosen (1994), four beliefs are associated with self-mutilation.

1. Self-mutilation is acceptable.
2. One's body and self are disgusting and deserving of punishment.
3. Action is needed to reduce unpleasant feelings.
4. Overt action is needed to communicate feelings to other people.

Throughout the counseling process, the social worker or other professional helps the client evaluate the validity of these beliefs and others that may be affecting their negative behaviors. See Table 6.1 for sample questions and strategies that could be used to challenge the aforementioned beliefs.

Table 6.1 Restructuring Thoughts for SMB

Core Belief:
Self-harm is acceptable.

Associated Negative Thoughts:
It's okay to cut, burn, etc. Other people cut, burn, etc.

Coping Thoughts:
It's not okay to cut, burn, etc. Just because other people cut, burn, etc., doesn't mean that I should.

Core Belief:
One's body and self are disgusting and deserving of punishment.

Associated Negative Thoughts:
I'm ugly.

Coping Thoughts:
Even though sometimes I feel ugly, I have pretty hair and nice eyes.

Most people feel ugly sometimes, but my mom and grandma tell me I'm beautiful.

Associated Negative Thoughts:
I'm fat.

Coping Thoughts:
Even though sometimes I feel fat, most people do at times, and I am an average weight.

The doctor isn't concerned about my weight, so I shouldn't be either.

(continued)

Table 6.1 *(Continued)*

(for an overweight person) Even though I am a little overweight now, I may not be overweight forever. My body is in my control and I can change it if I want to.

Core Belief:
Action is needed to reduce unpleasant feelings.

Associated Negative Thoughts:
No one likes me.

Coping Thoughts:
Even though not everybody likes me, lots of people do: my mom, grandma, friend A, B, & C, my youth pastor, sister/brother, etc.

Associated Negative Thoughts:
I'm alone.

Coping Thoughts:
That's not true! I have lots of people around that care about me: my mom, counselor, teacher, etc.

Associated Negative Thoughts:
I can't handle my emotions.

Coping Thoughts:
I can handle my emotions by doing coping strategies, problem solving, and changing my thinking.

Core Belief:
Self-harm is needed to communicate feelings to others.

Associated Negative Thoughts:
If I hurt myself, then others will pay more attention to me.

Coping Thoughts:
I do not need to hurt myself to get others to pay attention to me. I can ask (mom, teacher, counselor, sister, pastor, etc.) to talk if I am feeling stressed.

Another important component of cognitive therapy is to help the student develop a healthier set of coping skills. The mental health professional works with the client to develop activities such as journaling, listening to music, exercising, or engaging in relaxing activities when they experience the urge to cut. Case studies have illustrated that helping the client develop more proactive ways of dealing with concerns can reduce SMB. For example, Pipher (1994) worked with an adolescent female who engaged in self-mutilation when she became overwhelmed by societal problems such as HIV and homelessness. In addition to recommending journaling when the client is upset, the social worker or other school professional helped the adolescent to engage in activities that would address and sublimate her concerns. In this case study, the adolescent began to volunteer at a local soup kitchen, which in turn enabled the youth to feel as though she was contributing in a positive way to her concerns.

When developing coping strategies, it is often necessary to provide alternative behaviors that mimic the effects of self-mutilation without the accompanying physical harm (Alderman, 1997). This is especially important in the early phases of intervention when the adolescent may "crave" the physical effects of self-mutilation. The following are examples of replacement behaviors:

1. Have the adolescent wear a loose-fitting rubber band around his or her wrist and snap it when the urge to engage in self-mutilation occurs.
2. Have the adolescent tightly squeeze a piece of ice in the palm of his or her hand.
3. Have the adolescent submerge his or her arm in icy water.

Each of these behaviors will initiate the same physiological effects of self-mutilation but will not cause bodily harm. As counseling continues, the client should be encouraged to rely less on these strategies and engage in more active problem-solving solutions, such as journaling, engaging in social activities, and talking with others.

In summary, cognitive therapy appears to be a two-pronged approach to treating SMB. First, the intervention seeks to challenge maladaptive core beliefs that are promoting the self-mutilation behaviors. Second, the intervention provides the youth with alternative coping strategies and problem-solving skills.

Problem-Solving Therapy

Brief problem-solving therapy has shown promise in clinical trials as being efficacious in reducing the symptoms of SMB. Individuals who engage in SMB demonstrate specific deficits in their ability to effectively solve problems, and this type of therapy is helpful in teaching skills that may reduce their need to rely on maladaptive coping strategies. The primary goal of the therapy is to address the individual's current problems by identifying and defining them, deciding on goals, and using a stepwise approach to work toward their goals and improve the problems. The client is secondarily taught to practice and generalize these skills so that they can utilize them to address future problems. Problem-solving therapies have been effective not only in problem improvement but also in reducing the treated individuals' levels of depressions and hopelessness.

Emergency Card Provision

The provision of an emergency contact card in addition to other care has shown some positive effects for clients who engage in self-mutilation behaviors. The emergency card allows individuals to make an emergency contact when they have the desire to carry out the SMB. Although this strategy is not sufficient as a sole treatment, it has been helpful in reducing repetition of SMB in clinical trials.

Psychopharmacological Interventions

The U.S. Food and Drug Administration has not yet approved any psychopharmacological interventions for the treatment of SMB. Although there is a dearth of evidence-based research on this category of interventions, some medications have shown promise of efficacy in treating the symptoms of SMB in clinical trials, and many are used off-label with varying degrees of success. The selective serotonin reuptake inhibitors (SSRIs) are generally seen as the safest and most effective medications for treatment within this population. They are helpful in controlling the symptoms of impulsivity, depression, anxiety, irritability, and aggression with minimal side effects. Other classes of medications, such as mood stabilizers, opioid antagonists, beta-blockers, antipsychotics, benzodiazepines, monoamine oxidase inhibitors, and tricyclic antidepressants have shown some utility in treating the symptoms associated with SMB but should not be used as first-line treatments because of their increased negative side-effect profiles.

Tools and Practice Examples

Inquiring about self-harm behavior is a delicate undertaking. Because the behavior is contagious and is often learned from modeling, the social worker must be cautious not to give the child or adolescent ideas. Therefore, it may be important not to question directly about self-harm behavior if there is no prior evidence of it, especially when working with a population of children who are at risk of harming themselves.

The school social worker and other professionals working with a child or adolescent engaging in SMB should be first motivated to learn the function of the harming behavior. The social worker asks himself or herself, "What purpose is the self-harm serving?" Is the self-harmer seeking attention or pity from the social worker or someone else? If this is the root of the SMB, the self-harmer will usually be vocal about his or her self-harming behavior. The self-harmers may brag to peers, advertising the merits of cutting or burning oneself. The self-harmer also receives secondary gain by way of getting direct attention from the social worker or other professional after the incident(s), regular check-ins by school counselors, and possibly parental activation by way of increased attention and supervision. If this is the function of the SMB, the social worker may be curious about the child or adolescent's tendencies toward BPD. The school-based professionals would also be concerned about the spread of SMB to other students that the self-harmer encountered.

Is the self-harmer engaging in this behavior because he or she is trying to cope with stress by using a dangerous, maladaptive strategy? If this is the function of the SMB, the self-harmer may not choose to engage in self-harm if properly educated about other effective strategies. Viewing the child from a strengths-based perspective may help the social worker and other counselors when working with a child who harms because of an ineffective coping repertoire. In these cases, the professionals can perceive the self-harmer as someone who is trying to cope with his or her environment but has not learned better ways of doing so. With proper therapeutic intervention, the self-harmer can learn more adaptive ways of managing distress. Oftentimes, the SMB serves both of the functions described here. In these cases, treatment must address the attention function and coping function.

It is not uncommon for a child, especially a younger child, to be confused by his or her behavior. The child may be experiencing shame or guilt about the SMB on top of the angry or sad feelings which led to the self-harm.

Case Example

A 9-year-old child reported that she just woke up with all these scratches on her arm. She didn't know how it happened. Upon questioning, she insisted that she did not do it to herself, though the scratches were characteristic of self-harming behavior (vertical scratches breaking the skin about 2 to 3 inches in length).

With children like the one in the aforementioned example, it is not only necessary to conduct a thorough inquiry with the child but also necessary to inform the parents of the professional's clinical impressions. In such cases, parents should be educated about the signs of SMB and strongly encouraged to increase supervision of the child. Further recommendations to the parents might include organizing enjoyable activities for the child and parents to participate in together. The extra attention coupled with the fun activities would serve to facilitate the child's coping mechanisms.

Treatment

Cognitive-behavioral therapy focuses on first helping the child to describe the situation occurring when the child chose to self-harm. Next, the school social worker or other counselor helps the child recognize and identify negative emotions the child was feeling during that situation (before the self-harm) and the accompanying negative automatic thoughts leading to that emotion. Subsequent treatment is three pronged, consisting of enhancing the child's repertoire of coping skills, teaching problem-solving skills, and changing negative thinking. In addition, when working with a child who engages in self-harm, the helping professionals would be wise to complete a safety contract with the child. The safety contract should include people the child feels he or she can talk to when feeling the urge to self-harm (include phone numbers) and a coping plan with several coping strategies and positive coping thoughts listed. With some children, safer replacement behaviors, such as holding ice or snapping a rubber band on the wrist, can be added to the contract. Figure 6.1 presents the safety contract created for the child in the subsequent case study.

I, ------------------, agree not to harm myself. If I am having thoughts of harming myself I will do one or more of the following coping plans until I feel better:

1. Talk to someone (mom, dad, school counselor, youth pastor, aunt, grandmother). [include all phone numbers]
2. Play Playstation.
3. Play flute.
4. Run outside.
5. Listen to music.
6. Take a bubble bath.
7. Say my coping thoughts to myself:

   - "Who cares? Like it is cool to hang out with my sister's loser friends? Lots of other people think I'm cool, like my friends and my little sister."
   - "It is not my job to take care of my sister. I am 13 years old, and we have two parents whose job it is to take care of her."
   - "It can be hard to handle such a stressful situation, but I have lots of ideas of what I can do. If I do my coping plans, then I will feel better. Plus, I have handled lots of stressful situations in the past without hurting myself, such as my parents divorcing and moving to a new school."

1 understand the contract that I am signing and agree to follow it.

_____   _____
Child Signature   Parent Signature

_____
Social Worker/
Counselor

Date: --------------

Figure 6.1. Safety Contract.

Treatment should also be mindful of the possibility of more permanent or severe damage. In addition to scarring from burning or cutting, serious cuts could lead to infection or could hit a vein. There also may be social implications for those who engage in SMB. These children and adolescents are more isolated from peers because of their often secretive behavior. If the SMB becomes known, then they may be rejected by their peers who think the behavior is weird or fear that the self-harmer is dangerous.

Coping Skills
The child should be taught to replace the self-harm behavior with alternative coping behaviors that are engaging for the child. There are different categories

of coping skills, which are differentially effective for different negative emotions. For angry or irritable feelings, coping strategies that expend energy (e.g., running, biking, playing outside) can be highly effective. For worried or anxious feelings, coping strategies that induce relaxation (e.g., deep breathing, bubble bath) can be useful. Doing something to distract one's thinking (e.g., reading a book, surfing the Web, playing a game) is often helpful with many different negative emotions. The child should also be informed that different coping skills may work at different times, so it may be necessary to try a couple of coping strategies before one works to decrease the urge to self-harm.

Problem Solving

Problem solving focuses on actions the child can take to change situations that typically lead to the urge to self-harm. A few examples of problems that have been found to lead to self-harm in children and adolescents are fighting with siblings or parents, poor grades, family violence, parental substance abuse, and teasing by peers. It is important to emphasize that problem solving is only an option when the situation is one in which the child has some control (peer teasing). For instance, the child has no control over parental substance abuse. Problem solving can be taught concisely to children in a five-step process:

1. Identify the problem. What happened that provoked thoughts of self-harm?
2. Determine the goal. What does the child want to have happen?
3. Brainstorm plans. It is important to come up with at least five plans so the child can try a different plan if one does not work. Plans can include coping skills.
4. Guess the pros and cons of each plan and pick the best one(s). In this stage the child, guided by the professional, picks the best plan after estimating the pros and cons of each. Plans may be combined, too!
5. Praise yourself! The child should be encouraged for attempting to manage the situation without self-harm, even if the plan does not work out. Successful problem solvers are the ones who make an effort to remedy problems, even if the plans tried do not solve the problem.

A few suggestions for general problem-solving plans:

1. *Journaling.* Journaling is a cathartic process, which helps release negative emotions. With younger kids it may be helpful to structure the activity by giving them prompts (e.g., write down five things you are grateful for, write two good and two bad things that happened today, etc.).
2. *Increasing extracurricular activities.* Minimizing the time the child has to engage in SMB would be helpful.
3. *Drawing.* Like journaling, artistic expression is a way of coping and releasing emotion.
4. *Listening to music.* This is a fun and distracting activity and developmentally very appropriate for teens.

5. *Exercise.* As previously mentioned, exercise may be especially helpful for self-harmers. Aerobic activity releases endorphins, which are natural mood enhancers. Children may enjoy playing outside with friends, jumping rope, roller-blading, riding bikes, dancing, and playing sports. Adolescents may enjoy these activities in addition to organized exercise classes (e.g., aerobics, yoga).

Changing Negative Thinking

The third domain of intervention is working with self-harmers to identify and change negative thoughts associated with the SMB. As discussed previously, there are four core negative beliefs, each of which has commonly associated negative thoughts. The school social worker or other helper works with the child to restructure the negative beliefs into more positive, adaptive thoughts— thoughts that will not lead to SMB. Two techniques that are effective in restructuring negative thoughts are (1) developing a more positive explanation for the situation causing the negative thought and (2) discovering evidence that shows that the negative thought is not true.

Table 6.1 presents examples of the four core negative beliefs, commonly associated maladaptive thoughts, and potential replacement coping thoughts used in the restructuring process with adolescents who engage in SMB.

Case Example

Miranda is in sixth grade, the first year of middle school, and is 13 years old. She is Caucasian, with middle socioeconomic status, and has one older sister and one younger sister. Her parents are divorced, and recently she moved in with her father (she had been living with her mother), which resulted in changing to a middle school away from her elementary school friends. Miranda was retained in the third grade, thus is a year older and more physically developed than her peers. Miranda enjoys playing the flute in the school band and following the trends in Japanese animation. She was identified by her teachers and referred to the school counselor for exhibiting what was determined to be symptoms of depression. She had been attending weekly counseling sessions with the school social worker for 1 month when her mother called the school social worker reporting that she noticed an estimated 15 cuts, about 2 inches in length, on her daughter's arm.

Upon inquiry, Miranda reported that she had no specific thoughts about killing herself. Although she reported sometimes wishing she were dead when feeling angry, she would not act upon these feelings or thoughts. When asked more about the cutting, she described two incidents. One occurred at her mother's house and one at her father's house. At both times, other family members were at home. Miranda reported that the incidents were triggered by feelings of anger and confusion and that the cutting was a way to redirect her emotional pain and make her feel better. She said that the first time it did make her feel better but the second time it only helped a little bit, so she stopped doing it and tried a coping strategy (playing her flute), which worked better.

Sample Interview Addressing Self-Harming Behavior

The following text is an excerpt from a sample interview[i] with Miranda where the school social worker is inquiring about the self-harming behavior. In this example, the social worker has been informed by the child's parents that the child has engaged in self-harming behavior. The social worker has had an ongoing relationship with the child. The interview picks up after rapport has been established in that session.

S: I don't know if this is the case for you, but sometimes when children/ teens are feeling very stressed they may think about hurting themselves as a way to feel better. Has this happened to you?

C: Well, sort of.

S: Oh, I see. What happened?

C: My sister and I got in a huge fight on Saturday. She wanted to go hang out with her friends, who are kind of my friends too. I wanted to go with her but she didn't want me to go. She ended up leaving right in the middle of the fight and I didn't know what to do, so that's when it happened.

S: What did you do?

C: I took the scissors and made a few scratches.

S: Then what?

C: Then I played my flute.

S: Ok. So what emotion were you feeling when you picked up the scissors.

C: I don't know. I guess I was mad, and I didn't know what do to.

S: So, were you also confused?

C: Yeah, totally.

S: So, you were feeling mad and confused. What were you thinking? What thoughts were popping up in your head?

C: Well, that my sister thought I wasn't cool enough to hang out with her and her friends. I was also worried about her because sometimes she does bad things when she hangs out with her friends. So, I was thinking I should make sure I go with her so I can watch out for her but I couldn't get her to let me go along with her. I was thinking this is all too much and I couldn't handle it.

At this point the social worker has captured the triggering thoughts that cause the child to feel overwhelmed with emotion, which had led to the self-harming behavior. The school social worker could choose to help the child restructure any or all of these negative thoughts using cognitive restructuring techniques, but it was more important to use the session to develop a coping plan with the child so she could avoid cutting the next time she has these negative thoughts and emotions. It is essential that the social worker help the child recognize that these thoughts are triggers for her wanting to cut, so that if they occur again she can recognize that she needs to use other coping strategies.

S: You did a great job remembering the thoughts that you were having right before you picked up those scissors. Do you think you really wanted to hurt yourself or did you just want to feel better and not so overwhelmed?

C: I just didn't want to be so mad and mixed up about what to do.

S: That's understandable. It sounds like you were trying to cope with a difficult situation.

C: Yeah.

S: Well, let's see if we can come up with different and healthier ways to cope so that next time you are in a difficult and overwhelming situation you don't have to cut yourself.

It is important that the social worker empathize with the child's stress and desire to cope. It is also equally necessary for the child to agree that he or she really does not want to self-harm but just wants to feel better. Now the social worker and child are working toward the same goal.

S: So, in our previous meetings we have discussed a variety of coping strategies. Let's name them.

S & C: [Together they list five categories of coping strategies: do something fun and distracting, do something that uses energy, do something soothing and relaxing, talk to someone, and look at the situation in a more positive way. The social worker guides the child in identifying her favorite thing to do in each of the categories.]

S: Great! See you are already doing one of those coping strategies now by talking to me about this.

It is important to highlight the child's successes so that she feels a sense of competence in avoiding self-harming behavior. The social worker should continually look for sources of strength that the child already has (e.g., friends, family, an important hobby, a younger sibling, etc.), because it is through a person's strengths and resources that he or she is able to overcome challenges.

S: Now, let's look at this desire to cut as a problem that we can solve. To do that, we will work through the problem-solving steps. (The child has been taught the problem-solving procedure in past sessions.) So, what is the problem?

C: That I cut myself.

S: That's it. What is your goal?

C: Not to cut myself?

S: Right. And I think we figured out a minute ago that the goal is also to feel better. Do you agree?

C: Yeah.

S: So, what is the next step of problem solving?

C: Come up with plans?

S: Right! That's great. So, let's come up with our five plans. Remember that coping strategies can also be plans. What is one plan?

C: To talk to someone.

S: Good. Who would you talk to? [S & C list about five adults that the child could talk to. The child may want to add peers to the list, but it is important that if the child wants to talk specifically about the desire to cut, she should do so with supportive adults—not other children. If the child just wants to vent about feeling mad, sad, confused, etc., peers are good to talk to.] What is another plan?

C: I could play Playstation, or I could play my flute.

S: Yes, you could. Those are both fun and distracting activities. What else?

C: Run outside?

S: Yes! That is a great plan. Doing a coping strategy that uses energy, getting your heart rate up, is a particularly good plan when feeling mad. There are also chemicals in your brain that get released when you exercise. These chemicals are natural ways of feeling good.

It is important that if an energetic coping strategy is not on the child's list of plans, the social worker guides the child to make sure at least one is added. Replacing the cutting with another behavior that releases similar mood-enhancing chemicals can be particularly effective for reducing cutting.

S: We just need a couple more plans.

C: Listen to music? Take a bubble bath?

S: Great! Those are both soothing and relaxing activities. They may help you feel calmer if you are feeling intense negative emotions.

C: I can think something else?

S: Do you mean coming up with more positive thoughts?

C: Yeah.

S: Great idea! That is just what I was thinking, too. Let's come up with a few coping thoughts that would be really powerful for you. [S & C generate the following coping thoughts, which directly challenge the negative thoughts that led to the cutting behavior.]

S: So, as you know, the next step of problem solving is to guess how good each plan might be for achieving the goal of feeling better/not wanting to cut. Then, rank the plans in order from most effective to least effective. Remember, you can always combine plans or do more than one plan back-to-back.

Negative Thoughts	Coping Thoughts
"My sister would think I wasn't cool."	"Who cares?! Like it is cool to hang out with my sister's loser friends? Lots of other people think I'm cool, like my friends and my little sister."
"Something bad might happen to my sister."	"It is not my job to take care of my sister. I am 13 years old and we have two parents whose job it is to take care of her."
"This is too much for me to handle."	"It can be hard to handle such a stressful situation, but I have lots of ideas of what I can do. If I do my coping plans, then I will feel better. Plus, I have handled lots of stressful situations in the past without hurting myself, such as my parents divorcing and moving to a new school."

S: Ok, so now let's come up with a safety contract that will list all the great plans you came up with. [See Safety Contract.] Do you think you can agree to the contract?

C: Yeah.

S: Excellent. Then we will both sign it.

If the child is unsure whether he or she can agree to the contract, negotiate for the maximum number of days the child thinks the contract can be upheld. Upon the end of that time period, renegotiate as needed.

Key Points to Remember

- *Self-mutilation behavior* (SMB) is defined as the direct, deliberate, and repetitive destruction or alteration of body tissue, which results in minor to moderate injury, without conscious suicidal intent.
- SMB is NOT the same as a suicide attempt, but an estimated 10% of people who engage in an act of self-harm subsequently commit suicide.
- SMB is most often classified into the four broad categories of stereotypic, compulsive, major, and impulsive SMB.
- The prevalence rate of SMB has been difficult to determine but has been estimated at between 1.2% and 12% in adolescent samples.
- The functions of SMB in adolescents are most often to manage negative moods, as a response to negative beliefs, and to manage their social interactions.

- SMB is believed to have a neurochemical basis and is thought to produce euphoria, relieve tension, or reduce feelings of "numbness."
- Psychopathologies commonly associated with SMB are depression, eating disorders, personality disorders, and substance abuse.
- SMB is contagious.
- Treatment strategies that have shown promise in ameliorating the symptoms of SMB are cognitive and behavioral therapies, problem-solving therapy, emergency card provision, and psychopharmacological interventions.

Note

1. This sample interview is intended to serve only as a guide for clinicians. Each client is different, and the interview process needs to be tailored according to the client's specific needs.

Integrative, Solution-Oriented Approaches With Self-Harming Adolescents

Matthew D. Selekman

Getting Started

Adolescents today are growing up in a highly toxic, media-driven, consumerist culture and are struggling to cope with high levels of stress in all areas of their lives. Like a fast-acting pain killer, many adolescents report that self-harming behavior can offer them quick relief from emotional distress and other stressors in their lives. Several of my students have identified trying to fit in and keep up with their peers as the number one stressor they struggle with. Adolescents are plagued by "too-muchness," too many consumer choices, too many activities, too much homework, too many colleges to choose from, and so forth (Schwartz, 2004). Many of these youth are being hurried along into adulthood long before they are ready to assume these responsibilities. Their parents have overscheduled them in too many extracurricular activities and put a lot of pressure on them to pull in those high grades so that they can get into the *best* colleges possible!

Thanks to the power of media advertisements and the blatant biases of some of the major TV networks, teenagers are regularly seduced into believing that quick-fix solutions are the best way to manage stress and problems. Pharmaceutical companies are buying up more advertising time on major television network stations to market their wonder drugs for depression, anxiety, and attention deficit disorder. Several times a day, young people are being bombarded by violent images and receiving messages that the way to solve problems is to respond with aggression. In other forms of the media, teenagers see images of how certain alcoholic beverages can make them more "sexy," "social," and look "cool." They may observe their parents chain smoking or misusing alcohol and other drugs to relieve stress or to manage difficulties in their lives. Today's teenagers have learned a number of shortcuts for numbing away emotional distress and escaping from the demands of life, such as self-harming behavior. When adolescents cut or burn themselves, their bodies' immediately secrete endorphins into their bloodstream to quickly numb away the pain. Two commonalities that self-harming adolescents and adults share is that close to 70% of the students tend to experience relief from emotional distress after engaging in this behavior and tend to feel guilty and ashamed, and experience a downward swing in mood a few hours later (Favazza & Selekman, 2003). This, in turn, will often lead to thoughts of wanting to self-harm again to alleviate the emotional distress. Favazza (1998) also found that 50% of his students had concurrent difficulties with bulimia. See Chapter 6 for more information on the theory and research for this idea.

Many self-harming students report feeling emotionally disconnected and invalidated by their parents and, in some cases, their peers. One major cause of the family emotional disconnection process is high technology. Today, it is more important to be in chat rooms and playing Gameboys and computer games for hours on end than physically being with family and friends. Screens do not help develop or strengthen adolescents' social skills, and uphold family values, and make them more compassionate people. Many parents do not provide any guidelines around screen usage and then get upset with their kids for not wanting to spend time together as a family. In some cases, the parents are emotionally spent from their stressful jobs or are experiencing the perils of long-term unemployment and are just not available to provide emotional support to their kids. Unfortunately, this disconnection process may lead adolescents to seek refuge in a *second family* outside their own in the homes of unsavory peers who may be engaging in self-harming, substance-abusing, distressed eating, and other problematic behaviors (Selekman, 2006; Taffel & Blau, 2001). School social workers need to be sensitive to the role the aggravating factors have played in the development and maintenance of a student's self-harming behavior.

What We Know

The integrative, solution-oriented brief therapy approach to stopping self-harm, which is discussed in this chapter, comes out of the family systems and social construction orientations to counseling. Research is just beginning to emerge on how to stop adolescent self-harm. Many of the studies that have been conducted combined adolescents and adults in their samples (Favazza & Selekman, 2003; Santisteban, Muir, Mena, & Mitrani, 2003; Selekman, 2006; Favazza, 1998; Conterio & Lader, 1998). Santisteban et al. conducted a pilot study using their borderline adolescent family therapy model with adolescents who were diagnosed with borderline personality disorder and self-harming behavior. The researchers found that 70% of their sample was retained in therapy, and the clients rated their treatment experiences highly on alliance and satisfaction measures. This was one of the first attempts to study the effectiveness of family interventions with self-harming adolescents. Chapter 6 reviews other intervention studies.

What We Can Do

Over the past 10 years, I have been using an integrative solution-oriented brief therapy approach with self-harming adolescents (Favazza & Selekman, 2003; Selekman, 2005, 2006). Case studies and my own clinical experience indicate that solution-oriented, brief therapy (Berg & Miller, 1992; Berg & Steiner, 2003; De Shazer, 1991, 1988; O'Hanlon, 1987; O'Hanlon & Weiner-Davis, 1989) can produce good outcome results with at-risk adolescents. I have also found that it has its limitations with self-harming adolescent clients and could be improved and made more flexible by integrating compatible ideas from other therapeutic approaches, which can offer school social workers and other school-based counselors many more pathways for intervention. Two of the major limitations of the base model are (1) the strong emphasis on trying to engage self-harming adolescents as early in treatment as possible in *solution talk*, that is, eliciting from them mostly what is going *right* in their lives, which may block them from sharing their problem stories and further invalidate them, and (2) the fact that simply changing the adolescents' behavior or problem-maintaining family patterns may not alter their oppressive self-defeating thoughts and difficulties with mood management, which often contribute to the maintenance of the self-harming behavior. Many of these youth lack adequate cognitive and self-soothing skills. To address these limitations with the solution-oriented, brief therapy model, I integrated therapeutic ideas from narrative therapy (Epston, 1998; White, 1995; White & Epston, 1990), the collaborative language systems approach of Harry Goolishian and Harlene Anderson (Anderson, 1997; Anderson & Goolishian, 1988), positive psychology and cognitive therapy (Czikszentmihalyi, 1997; Fredrickson, 2002; Peterson & Seligman, 2004; Seligman, 2002; Seligman, Reivich, Jaycox, & Gillham, 1995), mindfulness meditation ideas (Bennett-Goleman 2001; Hanh, 2003, 2001), and the use of art therapy activities (Selekman, 2005, 2006, 1997).

Major Solution-Oriented Therapeutic Strategies and Experiments

In this section of the chapter, I present some of the major solution-oriented therapeutic strategies and experiments I regularly use with self-harming adolescents to empower them to achieve their treatment goals and resolve their difficulties. Since most school social workers and mental health counselors do not have access to students' parents because of their work schedules or have the luxury of doing family therapy sessions, I present only interventions that can be used with individual students.

Interviewing for Possibilities: Creating a Climate Ripe for Change in the First Session

When beginning the counseling process with new self-harming students, it is critical to take the time to elicit from them what their key strengths and resources and treatment expectations are. The students' strengths and resources can be channeled into their identified problem and goal areas to co-construct solutions. In our therapeutic conversations and with therapeutic experiment design and selection, we should use the clients' strengths, key words, beliefs, and metaphors connected to their major skill areas as much as possible to help foster a cooperative relationship with them. In addition, having the client talk about his or her strengths and resources triggers positive emotion, which can enhance his or her problem-solving capacities (Fredrickson, 2002).

In order to gain a better understanding of why the student gravitated toward self-harming behavior as a coping strategy, it is important to invite the student to share his or her story about how he or she discovered it, what specifically it does for the student, when and where is it most likely to occur, and what effect this behavior has on the significant others in his or her life. The students take the lead in determining the treatment goals they wish to work on, even if it has nothing to do with their self-harming behavior. Our job is to closely collaborate with them in negotiating small and doable behavioral goals.

Solution-Enhancement Experiment

This experiment is specifically designed for students to keep track on a daily basis of useful self-talk and coping strategies employed to avoid the urge or temptation to cut, burn, or engage in any other form of self-harming behavior (De Shazer, 1985; O'Hanlon & Weiner-Davis, 1989; Selekman, 2005, 2006). Once we identify with the student the specific self-talk tapes or coping strategies that help the most, we want to have him or her increase these solution-building patterns of thinking and doing.

Prediction Task

When the student reports that his or her self-harming behavior occurs on a random basis and he or she cannot identify key precipitants, the *prediction task* is the experiment of choice (De Shazer, 1991, 1988; Selekman, 2005). The student is instructed to predict the night before the next day whether or not a self-harming episode will occur. Later that next day, the student is instructed to try to identify all of the reasons why a self-harming episode did not occur. Similar to the solution-enhancement experiment, we want to increase the student's awareness of what works and to do more of it.

Pretend the Miracle Happened

When the student cannot identify any pretreatment changes or presently occurring exceptions (nonproblem behaviors, thoughts, or feelings), I like to offer the student the *pretend the miracle happened* experiment. For example, if a student has conflict with two of her teachers and she is failing those classes, I may have her pick 2 days over the next week to pretend to engage in the miracle-like behaviors she thinks they would like to see from her. While pretending to engage in the teachers' miracle behaviors for the student, she is to carefully notice how they respond to her. Oftentimes students are pleasantly surprised to see how people dramatically change when they alter their behavior. I have used this experiment with students who are experiencing peer difficulties as well.

Do Something Different

This experiment can be used in multiple ways in school settings. I offer it to students who are stuck engaging in unproductive ways of thinking or behaving that are further exacerbating their problem situations. For example, one of my former clients associated with a group of peers with whom she would be more than likely to share a razor blade. These peers were her best friends, and she was not ready or willing to sever her ties with them. As an experiment, I had her respond differently to them whenever they would encourage her to or begin to cut themselves around her. The client came up with three useful different ways of responding to them: leave the room in which the group self-harming behavior was occurring, change the topic when the idea of cutting was brought up, and raise the volume on the stereo and start dancing. According to my client, these creative strategies helped her successfully avoid the temptation to cut herself and at times would change her friends' behaviors as well. Similar to the pretend the miracle happened experiment, this change strategy can be used with clients who are experiencing difficulties with particular teachers.

Imaginary Feelings X-Ray Machine

When working with self-harming students who appear to have grave difficulty expressing their thoughts and feelings or have somatic complaints, I offer them the *imaginary feelings X-ray machine* experiment (Selekman, 1997, 2005, 2006). I have the student lie down on a long sheet of paper that has the durability of meat wrapping paper. The next step is to draw the outline of his or her body. I share with the adolescent to pretend that I have turned the X-ray machine on so I can see inside him or her what his or her feelings look like. The student is to draw pictures of what he or she thinks his or her feelings look like. The feelings can be depicted in scenarios from his or her life or in a symbol form. On a cautionary note, before making any interpretations about the meaning of any of the student's drawings, it is important to hear what the student has to say about his or her drawing. In addition, the social worker or counselor should present his or her interpretations in a tentative way, not as definitive explanations. Once adolescents draw out their feelings on paper, it is easier for them to talk about their unresolved issues and concerns. This art experiment is a wonderful exercise to use in adolescent groups.

Famous Guest Consultant Experiment

This playful thinking-out-of-the-box experiment taps clients' imagination powers to generate solutions for their difficulties (Selekman, 2005, 2006). I have students generate the list of three famous people that they have always admired or have been inspired by. These famous people can be historic figures, TV and movie celebrities, singers and groups, star athletes, artists, authors, and characters from popular books. I ask the students to pretend to put themselves in the heads of their selected famous people and think about how they would solve their problem or achieve their goal. Adolescents have a lot of fun with this experiment and often generate some very creative solutions with the help of their famous consultants.

Visualizing Movies of Success

This highly effective visualization tool can help disrupt the student's self-harming pattern of behavior (Selekman, 2005, 2006). The students have to close their eyes and capture a sparkling moment in their past where she they achieved or accomplished something that made them very proud of themselves. They have to apply all of their senses to the experience, including color and motion. I have the clients project this movie of success onto a screen in their head and watch it for 10–15 minutes with their eyes remaining closed. In order to get good at accessing their movies of success, I have students practice this visualization twice a day. What is interesting to note is that this exercise generates positive emotion in the person, which has been found to create a climate ripe for high-level problem solving (Fredrickson, 2002).

Mindfulness Meditation

Many self-harming students lack the capacity to soothe themselves when experiencing emotional distress. One effective tool we can teach them is *mindfulness meditation* (Bennett-Goleman, 2001; Hanh, 2001, 2003). There are many types of mindfulness meditations. Being mindful is one's ability to focus on one specific word, bodily sensation, or object and yet embrace or label everything that enters one's mind. I teach students about *mantras*, that is, a word or a line they can say to themselves for a designated period. If the word *mantra* is objectionable to the school or the client, another word can be used to describe the process. I also like to teach them food and sound meditation. Like the visualizing movies of success tool, it is helpful to practice meditating twice a day for 10–15 minutes at a time. Research indicates that mindfulness meditation can lower our breathing and heart rates, reduce our emotional reactivity when experiencing stress, and strengthen our self-awareness and concentration abilities (Bennett-Goleman, 2001; Selekman, 2006).

Interviewing the Problem

Interviewing the problem is a very creative narrative therapy experiment (Epston, 1998; Selekman, 2006) that can be used with students who have been oppressed by their self-harming behavior or other chronic difficulties for a long time. The social worker or counselor is to pretend to be a reporter for the *New York Times* newspaper covering a story on the students' identified problem (cutting, the attitude, bulimia, etc.). The students have to pretend to put themselves into the shoes of the problem and gain an inside-looking-out-perspective through its eyes and mind. Like a good reporter, the social worker or counselor needs to secure as many details as possible from the problem regarding its decision to enter the students' life; whether it is a friend or foe; how it has been helpful to the students; how it has wreaked havoc in the students' life; how it brainwashes the students; and what effect it has on their family members, peers, teachers, and other significant people in their life. The reporter can also ask the problem what the students and significant others do to thwart or frustrate it and what they do that works the most to undermine it when it is up to its tricks.

The power of this therapeutic experiment is that it helps liberate the students from the clutches of the problem and it can help them become more aware of the problem's tricks, so they can outsmart it when it is up to no good. Most adolescents like drama and find this experiment to be fun and insightful.

Habit Control Ritual

The habit control ritual was developed by Durrant and Coles (1991) to help empower the client, his or her parents, and involved helping professionals to conquer the externalized tyrannical problem. Once the student, the parents, the social worker, and concerned school staff have externalized the problem on the basis of the client's description of it or belief about it, as a team they can keep track on a daily basis of what they do to stand up to the problem and not allow it to get the best of them. They are also to keep track of the problem's victories over them. On a chart in the social worker's office, they can write down their effective coping and problem-solving strategies as well as the various ways the problem undermines their efforts by dividing them and promoting behavioral slips with the client. Like the interviewing-the-problem experiment, the client is liberated from the shackles of the problem and is free to pursue a new direction with his or her life. The parents' and school staff's original way of viewing the problem situation and interactions with the client can dramatically change as well.

Bringing in Peers and Inspirational Others

Some of the self-harming students we work with are struggling to cope with very stressful home situations. There may be destructive invalidating family interactions, or the parents may be emotionally disconnected from the students. They may have a few close and concerned friends at school who can be mobilized to provide added support for them. In addition, there may be a teacher or a coach who has taken a special interest in your client and is already providing advice and support to him or her. In fact, this *inspirational other* (Anthony, 1984; Selekman, 2006) may have a lot of creative ideas for helping your client. Bringing the concerned peers and the inspirational other into sessions as resources can help put in place a strong support system to help the client get to a better place. For example, Billy had a tendency to brutalize his body with pens and sharp items when peers at school would bully or tease him. For years, his older brother treated him the same way that the peers did at school. Billy's closest friend at school was Stacy and his inspirational other was his computer teacher Mr. Simon. With the permission of the school dean and Billy's parents, I was able to set up a crisis support team composed of the school social worker, Mr. Simon, Stacy, and another friend Phil. Whenever Billy would come to school emotionally distraught or he had been verbally abused by the bullies at school, an impromptu meeting would be arranged in the school social worker's office with the other crisis support team members to provide support and brainstorm solutions. With the help of the crisis support team, we completely eliminated Billy's self-harming behavior at school.

Constructive Management of Slips and Goal Maintenance

Self-harming students will experience inevitable slips throughout the course of intervention. Therefore, it is imperative that we prepare our students for how to constructively manage slips so that they do not escalate into prolonged relapsing and demoralizing crisis situations. First off, I like to normalize slips as signs that progress has already occurred, as teachers of wisdom, and as signs that more structure is needed during leisure times. It is important in second and subsequent sessions to ask consolidating questions (O'Hanlon & Weiner-Davis, 1989; Selekman, 2006) to help solidify the gains the student is making and how to quickly get back on track when slips occur. Some examples of consolidating questions are as follows:

- "What would you have to do to go backward at this point?"
- "What did you learn from that slip on Tuesday that you will put to good use the next time you are faced with a similar stressful situation?"
- "How were you able to stay on track on Monday?" "Wednesday?"
- "Let's say we got together in 3 weeks and you come in and tell me that you had a perfect vacation from counseling, what will you tell me you did to stay on track?"

Finally, we need to address any student concerns or intervene as early as possible if he or she reports that the goal maintenance situation is beginning to unravel. Otherwise, the student will feel like he or she has returned back to square one.

Tools and Practice Examples

Key Assessment Question to Ask Self-Harming Adolescents

- Where did you learn to cut or burn yourself?
- Has anyone significant in your past ever hurt you?
- What does the cutting/burning do for you?
- Are there any particular things that happen to you or thoughts you experience when you are more likely to cut/burn yourself?
- Are there any particular things that happen to you or thoughts and feelings that you experience when you are more likely to cut/burn yourself?
- What effect does your cutting/burning have on your relationship with your parents and/or siblings?
- How do your friends feel about your cutting/burning yourself?
- If you could put a voice to your cutting/burning habit, what would it say about you as a person and your situation?
- When you avoid the urge to cut/burn yourself, what do you tell yourself or do that works?

Taming the Mind: The Power of Mindful Meditation

The following techniques are effective in reducing self-harming behaviors among adolescents.

The Mantra

A mantra can be a word or a line that is meaningful to the adolescent. The word or line can be taken from one of their favorite tunes, books, or from their own unique self-generated self-talk tapes. The adolescent is to become so well acquainted with their mantra that it becomes a part of them. Adolescents should practice 10–12 minutes twice a day silently saying to themselves their mantras. The mantra can help center and soothe them when faced with stressors at home and at school.

Food Meditation

I like to use a raisin when doing this simple food meditation. A single raisin is placed in the adolescent's left palm. He or she is to carefully study the raisin's coloring, indentations/crevices, and shadowing around it for a few minutes. Then he or she is to slowly pick it up and roll it around on his or her fingertips, feeling its rugged texture for a few minutes. Next, he or she is to place the raisin in his or her mouth without biting down on it. This will trigger the salivation process. The adolescent should roll the raisin around his or her mouth with the use of his or her tongue. After doing this for a few minutes, he or she is to bite down on it, which will access the taste sensation. In his or her mind, the adolescent should describe its taste (sweet, tart, or sour). The adolescent is to slowly and finely chew up the raisin for a few minutes and not swallow it. Following this step, the adolescent should swallow it and pay attention to the sensations he or she experiences both while it is traveling down his or her esophagus and once it enters his or her stomach. The whole meditation process should last for approximately 10–12 minutes.

Sound Meditation

The adolescent is to find a nice quiet place to do this meditation. He or she is to sit comfortably in a chair or lie down on the floor. With eyes closed, the adolescent is to tune into all the various sounds he or she hears around him or her. While listening to each sound, the adolescent is not to get too attached to what he or she hears, just simply label it in his or her mind. This meditation should be done for 10–12 minutes.

Key Points to Remember

Self-harming students can be a challenge to work with. Their behavior can be quite intimidating for even the most seasoned of school social workers, counselors, and teachers. To further complicate matters, some of these adolescents' symptoms switch to bulimia, substance abuse, and sexual promiscuity as well. By following the guidelines provided here, social workers and other school professionals will be able to foster a cooperative relationship and create a context for change with self-harming students:

- Take the time to build a safe and trusting relationship.
- Provide plenty of room for the student to share his or her problem story.
- Go with whatever the student wishes to work on changing first.
- Utilize the student's key strengths and resources in presenting problem areas.
- Carefully match your intervention questions and experiments with the student's cooperative response patterns, strengths and resources, and treatment goals.
- Actively collaborate with concerned school staff.
- Involve the student's closest friends and inspirational others as resources in the counseling process.
- Normalize for the student the inevitability of future slips and teach tools for constructively managing them.

Effective Interventions for Students With Eating Disorders

Theresa J. Early

Getting Started

At times it seems as if every person in the United States is "on a diet." There are reports both of rising obesity rates among children and adults (see Chapter 9 for a discussion of this issue) and of unprecedented numbers of individuals attempting to stick to a diet that limits carbohydrates, fat, or both. Media images of the "ideal" body are unrealistic for most: too thin and out of proportion with real bodies, having a very small waist and overdeveloped chest. Within this context, many people, including children and youth, are dissatisfied with their bodies, and a small percentage of people develops eating disorders. Eating disorders are characterized by extreme obsessions with weight and eating, along with disordered behaviors around eating and weight control. Eating disorders are an important concern for school social workers and mental health personnel because these disorders often begin in adolescence. A number of school-based interventions aimed at prevention are described in the literature. In addition, professionals in the schools are in a position to notice eating disorders and assist with interventions, either through providing treatment or through supporting students who are participating in treatment in another setting. In this chapter, I discuss two types of eating disorders that are diagnosed in youth, anorexia nervosa and bulimia nervosa, and strategies of effective intervention based on the small amount of existing empirical evidence.

What We Know

Anorexia nervosa is more likely to begin during early adolescence, and bulimia nervosa is more likely to affect older adolescents and young adults, so both disorders may be seen in schools. Effective interventions have been identified for both bulimia nervosa and anorexia nervosa, but there is less empirical evidence regarding effective treatments for anorexia nervosa. Cognitive-behavioral therapy (CBT) has been identified as an effective treatment for bulimia nervosa through several randomized clinical trials (see, e.g., a review of 10 studies in Fairburn, Agras, & Wilson, 1992). Unfortunately, many of the studies of treatment effectiveness have been conducted with adults rather than among school-aged populations. However, several authors in the eating disorders field have described promising approaches that take into account adolescent development and the differences between anorexia nervosa and bulimia nervosa (Agras & Apple, 2002; Bowers, Evans, & Van Cleve, 1996; Lock, Le Grange, Agras, & Dare, 2001; Nicholls & Bryant-Waugh, 2003; Schmidt, 1998). In particular, Lock et al. (2001) have described a manualized family-based therapy approach for treatment of anorexia nervosa, which has evidence of effectiveness both as a primary treatment approach (Eisler et al., 2000) and following failure of other treatments (Sim, Sadowski, Whiteside, & Wells, 2004).

According to the standard diagnostic criteria used in mental health practice, anorexia nervosa is the refusal to maintain a (minimal) normal body weight along with intense fear of gaining weight or becoming fat (American Psychiatric Association, 2000). In addition, anorexia nervosa includes a distorted body image, including an unrealistic appraisal of body weight/shape and an overemphasis on body weight and shape for self-evaluation. Thus, individuals with anorexia nervosa may be dangerously underweight but believe themselves to be fat. In addition, they believe that their shape and weight are the most important aspects of themselves. Some individuals with anorexia nervosa also engage in binge-eating and/or purging behavior. Weight loss is achieved through some combination of extreme restriction in the amount and type of food eaten, excessive exercise, and purging (vomiting, using laxatives or diuretics). In females who have already begun to have menstrual cycles, amenorrhea also is part of anorexia nervosa.

Bulimia nervosa, on the other hand, is indicated by recurrent binge eating—eating a larger amount of food in a specific period than most people would eat and feeling a lack of control over eating during the binge episode. Individuals with bulimia nervosa usually weigh in a normal range because they also engage in behaviors that compensate for their overeating, such as purging, fasting, or excessive exercise. Bulimia nervosa shares with anorexia nervosa an overemphasis on body shape in evaluation of the self and extreme dissatisfaction with body weight and shape.

Anorexia nervosa is relatively rare, with an average prevalence rate of 0.3% in young females (Hoek & van Hoeken, 2003). Bulimia nervosa, although still rare, is more common than anorexia nervosa, having a prevalence of about 1% in young women (Hoek & van Hoeken, 2003). Although females are at much higher risk for these disorders, they do also occur in young males. Further, even though only a small number of young people with eating problems would meet the strict diagnostic criteria set out in the *DSM-IV-TR* (American Psychiatric Association, 2000), a greater number of youth experience many of the same obsessions with food and body image. These youth are at risk of developing eating disorders.

Risk factors include:

- dieting, especially repeated, unsuccessful dieting (for bulimia nervosa)
- perfectionism

- family history of eating disorder
- parental problems such as obesity or alcohol abuse
- critical comments by family members about the student's body weight or eating
- competitive involvement in gymnastics, swimming, wrestling, or ballet

The consequences of eating disorders in youth are serious and include dental problems, bone loss, osteoporosis, stunted growth, suicide, or death from excessive weight loss in extreme cases of anorexia nervosa. A number of other emotional disorders may also occur along with either anorexia or bulimia nervosa, including depression, anxiety disorders, obsessive-compulsive disorder, and personality disorders.

Although the cause of eating disorders is not conclusively known, one theory of causation is that a young person's insecurity becomes focused on his or her weight and shape. The energy of the person is directed toward strictly controlling food intake and weight. In anorexia nervosa, successful efforts at restricting food intake and losing weight may initially result in positive feedback from parents, teachers, or others whose opinions the youth values. The youth wants to continue to experience success, and control becomes its own reward. The young person continues to believe she or he is still too fat, even though the amount of weight lost may have been dramatic and dangerous. In bulimia nervosa, efforts to restrict food backfire into binge-eating episodes. The youth may try to control eating through restricting herself from certain foods (e.g., chocolate) for most of the day. The guilt and shame resulting from the loss of control, as well as intense fear of gaining weight, lead to attempts to compensate for the excess food, often through vomiting or taking excessive doses of laxatives.

What We Can Do

Tasks of the school social worker/counselor in relation to eating disorders include:

- offering effective prevention programs (discussed in Chapter 9 in this book)
- identification of youth with eating disorders
- assessment of the seriousness of a student's physical condition and enlisting the aid of parents
- if physical condition warrants, referring the student for medical treatment
- participating in cognitive-behavioral care after medical treatment *or* carrying out cognitive-behavioral intervention if medical treatment is not indicated

- assisting in monitoring medication effectiveness and side effects, if pharmacological treatment is being given
- providing support for students who are receiving treatment in other settings

Identifying Youth With Eating Disorders

- Physical signs include significant changes in weight, especially weight loss; failure to gain weight or height expected for the age and stage of development; and delayed or disrupted puberty. In anorexia, abnormal hair growth (soft, downy) may be present on the face or back.
- Behavioral signs include limited food intake, either in terms of energy quality or nutrient range; excessive or irregular food intake.
- Social signs may include social isolation and withdrawal from friends and activities.

Other school personnel also are in a position to identify youth with eating disorders. Teachers and coaches, in particular, may have more regular, ongoing contact with students than do school social workers or counselors. Therefore, it is important for the school mental health professional to be a resource for other school personnel in regard to identifying and responding to signs of eating disorders in students.

Assessing Seriousness of Physical Condition

A diagnosis of anorexia nervosa requires that weight be 85% of normal weight for height and developmental stage (or less) and in postmenarche females, amenorrhea of at least three cycles. If a student meets these criteria, the school social worker should refer the youth for a medical checkup. Hospitalization may be necessary if the youth is 75%–80% of expected body weight. Bulimia nervosa has fewer potential medical complications unless the youth is heavily abusing laxatives or diuretics, in which case, electrolyte levels may become out of balance and cause rapid changes in blood pressure and/or pulse rate. If in doubt, the social worker should refer the student for a medical checkup.

Enlisting the Aid of Parents

The involvement and support of parents is important in treating many emotional and behavioral disorders in children and youth. In treating eating disorders, family support is critical. Although there may be family dynamics that play into a youth's eating disorder, it is important to avoid blaming parents for their child's eating disorder. Family therapy to improve expression of emotions and general communication may be helpful in treating a youth's eating disorder. In family-based therapy for eating disorders, parents are specifically put in charge of refeeding their child; family relationships are renegotiated to increase parental monitoring for prevention of binge/purge behaviors; and youth are assisted with normal adolescent development (separation and individuation) (Lock et al., 2001).

Steps in Cognitive-Behavioral Intervention for Eating Disorders

The primary targets of CBT intervention for bulimia nervosa and anorexia nervosa are (1) modifying the beliefs and attitudes that support the importance of body shape and weight; and (2) normalizing eating. CBT for eating disorders, manualized initially by Fairburn, Marcus, and Wilson (1993) and more recently by Agras and Apple (1997), relies on a variety of behavioral and cognitive strategies. The treatment is problem oriented, focused on the present and future, and proceeds (for bulimia nervosa) over 19 sessions in three stages.

Stage 1. The goal of the first stage is to normalize eating. During the first session, the mental health professional orients the student to the goals and processes of therapy. The youth must be willing to play an active role in therapy and must develop confidence in the mental health professional and the cognitive-behavioral approach. Illustrating the cognitive model of eating disorders, the mental health professional helps the student to draw connections between his or her own situation and the links among emotions, dietary restrictions, binge eating, and purging. The mental health professional emphasizes the importance of regular meals—three meals and two snacks daily, going no more than 3–4 hours (while awake) without eating—highlighting how hunger and cravings from strict dieting lead to binge eating and purging. Accurate information about food, nutrition, and weight regulation is provided. The mental health professional will ask the youth to make one change (e.g., eat something in the morning if breakfast is usually skipped).

Self-monitoring is an important strategy in cognitive-behavioral interventions. During the first session, the mental health professional teaches the youth to use the Daily Food Diary (see Figure 8.1). This form is used to track what the youth eats, when, and how much, and various aspects of the context of eating, such as the location and associated thoughts and feelings about each episode of eating. The youth also classifies each episode as a meal, snack, or binge and records purging behavior. The purpose of keeping the food record is to identify eating episodes that are handled appropriately as well as patterns of problems and the factors that contribute to them. The record also can be used to track progress over time.

Stage 2. Once the student is eating more regularly and having fewer episodes of binge eating and purging, the treatment moves on to more cognitive aspects. The Daily Food Diary has probably already turned up some of the triggers of problematic situations, thoughts, and emotions. One of the basic tenets of CBT is that individuals commit thinking errors, using faulty logic. The interpretation of events resulting from these errors causes negative emotions. To relieve negative emotions, then, the youth engages in binge eating, purging, or

Name _____   Day _____   Date _____

Time	Type & Amount Food/Beverage	Place	Snack (S) Meal (M) Binge (B)	Purge (V/L)	Situation

Figure 8.1. Daily Food Diary.

other control mechanisms in order to feel better (less anxious, for example). The mental health professional now teaches the student to identify and challenge the dysfunctional thoughts that are influencing his or her emotions and behavior. A method for challenging dysfunctional thoughts involves using the Daily Record of Dysfunctional Thoughts (see Figure 8.2). From the first session on, the mental health professional should help the student to clarify the difference between thoughts and emotions to model the identification of emotions and the uncovering of automatic thoughts. The mental health professional then helps the student identify more rational thoughts to substitute for the dysfunctional thoughts.

This stage also includes behavioral experiments through which the student actively challenges his or her dysfunctional thoughts. Usually, the youth is convinced that there are certain foods that he or she just cannot eat because to

Name _____   Day _____   Date _____

Situation	Emotions	Automatic Thoughts	Rational Response

Figure 8.2. Daily Record of Dysfunctional Thoughts.

have even a small amount would have a disastrous effect on his or her weight or shape. The intervention uses the Feared Foods List (see Figure 8.3) to identify these foods and rank them in terms of difficulty on a scale of 1–4, with 1 being the easiest to handle. The goal here is to experiment with adding a moderate-sized portion of one or more of these foods, starting with the easiest ones to the eating plan once per week or every other week. The youth should record his or her reactions to consuming the feared food in his or her Daily Food Diary and process dysfunctional thoughts that arise.

Stage 3. The final stage of treatment is to create a maintenance plan. The mental health professional and student should brainstorm and problem solve about upcoming events and situations that are high risk for the student. The student should be prepared for a relapse of some of the disordered eating

1. Food or beverage	Rank Difficulty (1 = easiest to deal with)
------------------------------------	1 2 3 4
------------------------------------	1 2 3 4
------------------------------------	1 2 3 4
------------------------------------	1 2 3 4
------------------------------------	1 2 3 4
------------------------------------	1 2 3 4
------------------------------------	1 2 3 4
------------------------------------	1 2 3 4
------------------------------------	1 2 3 4
------------------------------------	1 2 3 4
------------------------------------	1 2 3 4

2. Select one or more of the food items rated "1." Describe a plan for consuming moderate-sized portions each week or every other week. Describe your reaction in your Daily food Diary.

Food/Beverage	Amount in a Moderate Portion	How Often to Consume

Figure 8.3. Feared Foods List.

behaviors and have plans in place for what he or she will do. The student should write out plans of what he or she will do if/when relapse occurs. The plan should be specific, including making reframing statements to himself or herself ("I have binged on fatty food today, but that does not mean that I am back to having an eating disorder") and returning to practicing the cognitive and behavioral strategies that were effective. The goal is for the student to be able to apply the tools he or she has learned before a short-term relapse gets out of hand and becomes a longer-term problem.

Monitoring Medication Effects and Side Effects
Table 8.I lists some medications that may be used in treatment of anorexia nervosa and bulimia nervosa. Medications usually would be used in conjunction with therapy. Antidepressant medications combined with CBT seem to be an effective combination (Halmi, 2003).

If a student is receiving treatment that includes medication for an eating disorder, the school social worker or mental health professional should watch for the

Table 8.1 Medications Used in Treatment of Eating Disorders

Medication/Source:
Fluoxetine (Prozac) or other SSRIs (Halmi, 2003)

Disorder:
Anorexia nervosa

When Used:
Following some weight restoration

Symptoms Targeted:
Prevent relapse; reduce depression, anxiety, and obsessive-compulsive symptoms

Side Effects:
Nervousness, difficulty falling asleep or staying asleep, upset stomach, dry mouth, sore throat, drowsiness, weakness, shaking of hands

Medication/Source:
Fluoxetine (Prozac) or other SSRIs (Halmi, 2003)

Disorder:
Bulimia nervosa

When Used:
During treatment
Symptoms Targeted:
Reduce binge eating; improve mood; reduce preoccupation with shape and weight

When Used:
Aftercare
Symptoms Targeted:
Prevent relapse

Side Effects:
Nervousness, difficulty falling asleep or staying asleep, upset stomach, dry mouth, sore throat, drowsiness, weakness, shaking of hands

Medication/Source:
Topiramate (anticonvulsant) (Kotwal, McElroy, & Malhotra, 2003)

Disorder:
Bulimia nervosa

When Used:
During treatment

Symptoms Targeted:
Reduce binge eating and purging

Side Effects:
Fatigue, flu-like symptoms, prickling or tingling or decreased tactile sensations of the skin, rare but serious side effects include kidney problems, eye problems (acute myopia and acute angle-closure glaucoma)

intended effects and side effects, as listed in Table 8.1, and communicate these observations to parents and/or medical personnel treating the student.

Practice Example

Tina was referred to the school social worker when her homeroom teacher noticed that Tina was throwing up in the bathroom after lunch. The teacher asked Tina whether she was sick and needed to go home, and Tina's hesitation led the teacher to walk Tina to the social worker's office. In tears, Tina admitted to the social worker that she made herself vomit because she didn't want to gain weight. After a conference later in the week with Tina's mother, the social worker began meeting with Tina during a free period.

The social worker learned that Tina was the youngest child of four in the family. Growing up, she idolized her older sister, Judy. Tina had medical problems from birth and was babied a great deal by her parents and her older siblings. One day when Tina was about 13 years old, Judy remarked on Tina's shape, saying teasingly that she was "getting to be a little fatty." Tina was hurt—and enraged—and vowed to herself to "show her!" Although she was actually a normal weight, Tina began on a diet immediately. For the next several weeks, she followed a pattern of eating little but thinking about food all the time. Initially she lost weight, but after a couple of months, one day she was so hungry after school that she stopped on the way home and bought a box of chocolate-covered doughnuts. She meant to eat one, but soon realized she had eaten the whole box. Then she stopped at another store and bought a quart of milk. She drank the whole quart and then felt sick. This pattern continued for several days. Tina grew more and more concerned about her weight and began to make herself vomit after the doughnuts and milk.

Stage 1. The social worker got Tina to describe her eating pattern, which consisted of no breakfast, plain lettuce at lunch, then a binge on doughnuts, milk, roasted chicken, ice cream, and other foods on the way home. Tina would vomit after the binge, then eat dinner in her room, and vomit again before bedtime. The social worker explained the food record and the goal of eating something every 3–4 hours. Tina was alarmed that eating this much would make her weight go up. The social worker explained that eating a normal amount of food spread out over the day should result in a stable weight and that Tina's pattern, even though her intent was to lose weight through purging the food she eats, actually may be resulting in weight gain. Her strict restriction of food during the day leads to the cravings she experiences and gives in to on the way home. She feels guilty until she purges. The social worker explained that even though Tina is vomiting, it is likely that she is not able to get rid of all of the calories in the food she has consumed. Tina agreed to try to eat a small bowl of cereal with milk and half of a banana for breakfast.

The next week, Tina reported eating breakfast as planned and adding two crackers to her salad at lunch. However, she was still binge eating on doughnuts and/or roasted chicken on the way home and purging. She reported that she meant to eat only half of the doughnuts, but was unable to stop. She was able to then eat a normal amount for dinner and not purge. She worried about her weight, which was up 2 pounds from the last week. The social worker explained that weight fluctuates as much as several pounds up or down per day, often depending on water retention (e.g., from where she is in her menstrual cycle or from eating a great deal of salty food). Pointing out to Tina that it is a long time between breakfast and the end of the school day, with only a small amount of food that amounts to anything in between, she suggested that Tina add something to her lunch. Tina agreed to add cheese and crackers and tomato to her plain lettuce.

Stage 2. As Tina adopted a more regular meal and snack schedule, she was able to avoid binge eating on the way home on most days. When she got a bad grade on a test, though, she binged on doughnuts once again. At this point, the intervention moved on to the thoughts and emotions that were associated with her eating disorder. All along, the social worker had tried to help Tina to recognize her emotions. Like many other people, Tina is not always able to label how she is feeling, confusing thoughts and feelings. In discussing the test grade, Tina said, "I feel like I'll never be able to get into a good college with these grades." The social worker responded, "You think your grades may keep you from getting into a good college, and you feel scared or sad about that." Tina acknowledged that she feels scared; she was afraid she will disappoint her parents. The social worker introduced the Daily Record of Dysfunctional Thoughts (Figure 8.2) and helped Tina to fill it out with this example:

SW: The situation is getting a bad grade on a test. Your emotions—how you feel—is scared. What is it that you think automatically about this?

Tina: My parents will think I'm not smart enough to go to a good college.

SW: Okay, let's come up with a more rational thought. Do you really think that one test grade will keep you out of a good college?

Tina: No, I guess not.

SW: Is this bad grade what you usually get on tests?

Tina: No, I usually do much better.

SW: What was the grade?

Tina: I only got 85%.

SW: Aha, now I see. How about this for a more rational response: "Even though I got a B on the test, it is just one test. A few B's won't hurt my overall GPA anyway."

Tina: Okay, but my parents are still going to be upset.

SW: What will happen because they are upset about the grade?

Tina: I guess they will still love me.

Stage 3. Tina accomplished a great deal in treatment. She was eating regular meals and snacks, rarely binge eating, knew what was likely to trigger a binge-eating episode, and had begun to exercise more regularly. There were only a couple of sessions left, and school would be out soon for summer. Tina and the social worker were thinking about high-risk situations that might come up for Tina in the near future. Tina would be going away to band camp in July and had identified that as a potentially risky time. Tina decided to begin keeping the food diary again a week before she leaves for camp. In this way, she will be able to monitor her emotions and eating while she is away. If she begins to have problems sticking to a regular meal schedule or is tempted to binge, she will work on a more rational response to what she is feeling and thinking. If she does binge and/or purge while she is away, she will remind herself that she can stop again when she gets home.

Key Points to Remember

- Eating disorders (meeting full diagnostic criteria) are fairly rare but may have serious consequences. School personnel should be attuned to extreme weight loss and other signs of disordered eating behavior. A greater number of students may have disturbed eating behaviors that may later lead to a full-blown eating disorder.
- Individuals with anorexia nervosa are more likely to have medical complications. If anorexia nervosa is suspected, there should probably be a referral for a medical examination.
- Bulimia nervosa in particular is amenable to treatment with a cognitive-behavioral intervention. The treatment that is described here and in the treatment manuals referenced consists of 19 sessions in three stages.
- The first stage of treatment emphasizes restoring a normal eating pattern of three meals and two snacks per day.
- Stage 2 of treatment addresses the distorted thinking and emotions that lead to and maintain eating disorders.
- Stage 3 plans for relapse prevention.
- Medications are sometimes used along with therapy during treatment or afterward for relapse prevention.

Effective Management of Obesity for School Children

Reshma B. Naidoo

Getting Started

The incidence and prevalence of obesity in the United States has increased rapidly since the 1980s. Estimates from studies conducted in 2002 indicate that approximately 64.5% of the U.S. population is overweight, with 30.5% being obese (Ogden, Flegal, Carroll, & Johnson, 2002). Estimates also indicate that 15% of school-aged children are obese (National Center for Health Statistics, 1999; Flegal, Carroll, Ogden, & Johnson, 2002). This increase in obesity has been attributed to a lack of physical activity combined with unhealthy eating patterns.

Overweight children are more likely to become overweight adolescents, who in turn are more likely to become overweight adults (Dietz, 1991; Serdula et al., 1993). Overweight and obese individuals are at increased risk for several significant health and psychosocial problems (see Table 9.1) (Epstein, Wisniewski, & Weng, 1994). Given the range of problems experienced by obese individuals, effective management of obesity in a school-aged population has to be addressed across multiple environments that include the home and school.

Body mass index (BMI) is a commonly used indicator of obesity in which weight (in kilograms) is divided by the square of height (in meters). A BMI of 25 or greater is defined as overweight and a BMI of 30 or greater is defined as obese (Bellizzi & Dietz, 1999).

What We Know

Almost all children are enrolled in schools, giving us the best opportunity to introduce obesity management and prevention programs that can influence the long-term health and well-being of children. Teaching children effective ways to control their weight provides them with a foundation that they can use to maintain healthy body weights into adulthood. Furthermore, school-based programs have the potential to effect behaviors that track into adulthood (Lytle, Kelder, Perry, & Klepp, 1995).

Most school-based programs have focused on obesity prevention and weight control (Carter, Wiecha, Peterson, & Gortmaker, 2001; CATCH, 2003; Cheung, Gortmaker, & Dart, 2001; Gortmaker et al., 1999). There is a paucity of evidence-based obesity management programs or guidelines for children

Table 9.1 Health and Psychosocial Problems Associated With Obesity

Psychosocial Problems	Health Problems	
Victims of bullying	Coronary heart disease	Cancers
Lower social status	High blood pressure	Gallbladder disease
Poorer self-esteem	Angina pectoris	Stroke
Young adult eating disorders	Congestive heart failure	Gout
Reduced quality of life	High blood cholesterol	Eye disorders
Distorted body image	Type II diabetes	Osteoarthritis
Depression	Hyperinsulinemia	Sleep apnea or sleep disorders
Psychosocial ailments	Insulin resistance	
Loneliness	Glucose intolerance	
	Poor reproductive health	
	Bladder control problems (stress incontinence)	

Source: Table 9.1 was compiled by synthesizing information from several sources that included Epstein, L. H., Wisniewski, L., & Weng, R. (1994). Child and parent psychological problems influence child weight control. *Obesity Research, 2*, 509–515. National Institutes of Health (1998). *Clinical guidelines on the identification, evaluation, and treatment of overweight and obesity in adults*. Bethesda, MD: Department of Health and Human Services, National Institutes of Health, National Heart, Lung, and Blood Institute. Stunkard, A. J., & Wadden, T. A. (Eds.). 1993. *Obesity: Theory and therapy* (2nd ed.). New York: Raven Press.

(Barlow & Dietz, 1998). Consequently, a consensual agreement between experts in the field resulted in the development of a list of guidelines for obesity management programs at schools (Barlow & Dietz, 1998). The major emphases of these guidelines are presented in Table 9.2.

There are several good school-based interventions that focus on decreasing the major identified risk factors for obesity and fostering a healthy lifestyle such as *CATCH* (CATCH, 2003), *Eat Well and Keep Moving* (Cheung, Gortmaker, & Dart, 2001), and *Planet Health* (Carter, Wiecha, Peterson, & Gortmaker, 2001). The goal of these programs is to teach children healthy lifestyle habits. They focus on reducing obesity, increasing physical activity, and fostering positive dietary habits. Programs range from 8 weeks to several school years in duration. However, there is a paucity of school-based individual and/or small group

Table 9.2 Goals for Treating Childhood Obesity

- Dietary modifications:
  - −Reduce intake of dietary fat
  - −Increase the intake of fruits and vegetables
  - −Decrease soda consumption
- Increase physical activity
- Decrease television, computer, and video game time

Source: Information extracted from Barlow, S. E., & Dietz, W. H. (1998). Obesity evaluation and treatment: Expert committee recommendations. Pediatrics, 102, p. E29. Retrieved November 2004 from http://www.pediatrics.org/cgi/content/full/102/3/e29http://www.pediatrics.org/cgi/content/full/102/3/e29

programs that address the treatment and interventions of obesity management. A structured school-based weight loss program would help the child to decrease his or her percentage overweight by fostering a healthy lifestyle. The advantage of a school-based program is that children are (a) able to lose weight and (b) maintain their weight loss into adulthood (Knip & Nuutinen, 1993). Furthermore, children who have been placed on weight loss programs are better at keeping the weight off compared to adults, even 10 years after the completion of the weight loss program (Epstein, Valoski, Wing, & McCurley, 1994; Epstein, Valoski, Kalarchian, & McCurley, 1995).

Although there has been considerable research into treatment programs since the 1970s, there is no structured school-based obesity management intervention. This intervention is based on the best practices driven by research in the field. Major research findings used to develop this program are summarized in Table 9.3.

What We Can Do

The Obesity Management Program (OMP) is a school-based weight loss and behavioral modification program for overweight and obese individuals. The OMP is an individual therapy, and the school-based segment can be modified for groups. This multipronged program focuses on developing a healthy lifestyle that facilitates weight loss. Skills are introduced gradually over a 14-week period (see Table 9.4) and are reinforced at home and school until the child/adolescent is able to practice them without assistance. The success of the program depends upon home–school collaboration and requires active involvement of the family. Homework is assigned at the end of each weekly session to reinforce and practice new skills. Practicing skills and the completion of homework is essential for the success of the program.

Table 9.3 Well-Established Treatments and Supporting Studies	
Established Treatment Modality	*Supporting Studies*
Children-centered programs have long-term benefits	Epstein, Valoski, Wing, & McCurley, 1994; Epstein, Valoski, Kalarchian, & McCurley, 1995; Knip & Nuutinen, 1993; Lytle, Kelder, Perry, & Klepp, 1995
Increased lifestyle activity is more efficacious and enduring than structured exercise programs	Epstein, Wing, Koeske, Ossip, & Beck, 1982; Epstein et al., 1994
Gradually scheduled programs provide more support for behavior modification programs	Senediak & Spence, 1985; Rees, 1990
Rewards for increasing desired or decreasing undesired behaviors are more effective reinforcers than punishment or disincentives	Coates, Jeffery, Slinkard, Killen, & Danaher, 1982; Epstein, Valoski, Vara, et al., 1995
Multimodal treatment strategies that include the family and school are more effective than unitary programs	Brownell, Kelman, & Stunkard, 1983; Epstein, Wing, Koeske, Andrasik, & Ossip, 1981; Epstein , Wing, Steranchak, Dickson, & Michelson, 1980; Epstein, Valoski, Wing, & McCurley, 1990; CATCH, 2003; Cheung et al., 2001; Carter et al., 2001; Gortmaker et al., 1999; Lytle et al., 1995
Systemic approach to behavior modification	Goetz & Caron, 1999; Raue et al., 1993; Golan et al., 1998
Mentoring and support	Buckley & Zimmermann, 2003
24-hour recall records	Baxter & Thompson, 2002; Armstrong et al., 2000.

Tools and Practice Examples

Practice Examples

Lisa had entered the 6th grade at middle school. After the first 6 weeks, Ms. Halferty, her homeroom teacher, noticed that although Lisa was making adequate academic progress, maintaining an A/B average, she had difficulty adjusting to middle school. Lisa had low self-esteem, was very self-conscious, and often sat by herself. Ms. Halferty was concerned about Lisa's isolation from her peers and attributed Lisa's social difficulties to her obesity. Lisa had

Table 9.4 Obesity Management Program: Weekly Goals

Week	Objective
Week 1 *Town* *meeting*	1. Establishing a family–child–school collaboration in weight management a. Rationale for program b. The role of the family–school collaboration c. Overview of the program, duration, and procedure d. Cost of the program e. Family commitment and contract • U.S. obesity trends 1985 to 2002 are available at: http://www.cdc.gov/nccdphp/dnpa/obesity/trend/maps/index.htm • Parent handout: *Obesity in children: A prevention guide for parents* available at: www.nasponline.org/pdf/Obesity.pdf • Parent handout: *Obesity in children and teens:* A parent information sheet available at: http://www.aacap.org/publications/factsfam/79.htm
Week 2 *Getting* *started*	1. Outlining the program with the child 2. Establishing baselines 3. Completing forms 4. Homework—completion of daily record sheets for the week • BMI calculators are available at: www.cdc.gov/nccdphp/dnpa/bmi/calc-bmi.htm
Week 3 *On your* *marks…*	1. Introduction of the weekly weigh-in 2. Understanding baselines and plotting charts a. BMI b. Television viewing patterns c. Physical activity patterns d. Foods chart—what I am eating 3. Television and advertising—how it affects our eating patterns 4. Introduce the "5-a-day program" 5. Homework—completion of daily record sheets for the week. • Copies of the 5-a-day program, facts of the day, and interesting recipes can be obtained at http://www.cdc.gov/nccdphp/dnpa/5aday/index.htm
Week 4 *Get set…*	1. Weekly weigh-in 2. Checking in: diet, television, and physical activity logs. Plot your progress 3. What do I do when I watch TV? 4. Reading food labels 5. Homework • A Web site with information to help children learn how to read food labels: http://kidshealth.org/kid/stay_healthy/food/labels.html

(continued)

Week	Objective

Table 9.4 *(Continued)*

Week	Objective
Week 5 Go!	1. Weekly weigh in 2. Checking in: diet, television, and physical activity logs. Plot your progress 3. The food pyramid and what that means 4. How to increase my physical activity 5. Homework • A Web site with information to help children learn about the food pyramid: http://kidshealth.org/kid/stay_healthy/food/pyramid.html • *The Food Guide Pyramid* can help families make healthy eating choices and is available from the Center for Nutrition Policy and Promotion, 703–305-7600 and at www.usda.gov/cnpp/pyrabklt.pdf
Week 6 Pacing	1. Weekly weigh-in 2. Checking in: diet, television, and physical activity logs. Plot your progress 3. Good foods versus bad foods—a review 4. Stoplight diet 5. Homework • Peer support, food logs, and weigh-ins help to keep the child on track • *The Stoplight Diet for Children: An Eight-Week Program for Parents and Children* (1988) by Leonard Epstein and Sally Squires, published by Little Brown & Company, is a comprehensive guide.

The Stoplight Diet: A brief primer

This is a parent–child team effort developed by Dr. Leonard Epstein.
* Foods are linked to the three signals on a traffic light:
  • High-calorie foods that contain fats, oils, and simple sugars, like soda and cookies, are "red" and should rarely be eaten.
  • Moderate-calorie foods, like cereal, dairy products, and meat are "yellow" and should be eaten with caution.
  • "Green" foods, which include most vegetables, fruits, breads, and grains get the go-ahead.
* This diet is aimed at changing what different foods mean, changing the meaning of snacks from red to healthy "green foods."
  • A useful parent resource on the health consequences of obesity is: http://diabetes.about.com/cs/kidsanddiabetes/l/blNIHkidsweight.htm

(continued)

Week	Objective
Table 9.4 (Continued)	
Week 7 *Steady* *does it*	1. Weekly weigh-in 2. Checking in: diet, television, and physical activity logs. Plot your progress 3. Increasing your physical activity—walk whenever you can 4. Homework • Resources for planning a "kids walk to school day" that include parent handouts for alternative activities: http://www.cdc.gov/nccdphp/dnpa/kidswalk/resources.htm#Train
Week 8 *Looking* *good!*	1. Weekly weigh-in 2. Checking in: diet, television, and physical activity logs. Plot your progress 3. Reviewing the stoplight diet 4. Progress: Calculating my BMI 5. How much television am I watching? 6. Planning a "turn your television off" week 7. Homework • A good resource for parents: Obesity and television fact sheet can be obtained at: http://www.mediafamily.org/facts/facts_tvandobchild_ print. shtml • Reducing TV time: Guidelines for running the "turn your television off week" program as well as important dates and activities: http://www.tvturnoff.org/index.htm
Week 9 *Keep on* *moving!*	1. Weekly weigh-in 2. Checking in: diet, television, and physical activity logs. Plot your progress 3. Brainstorm ways to increase your activity when you are sitting 4. Reviewing how the "turn your TV off week" will be run 5. Homework—"turn your TV off week" • A Web site for alternative activities to do with the "extra" time: http://www.tvturnoff.org/action.htm
Week 10 *Paying off!*	1. Weekly weigh-in 2. Checking in: diet, television, and physical activity logs. Plot your progress 3. Reevaluation of program a. How much of progress have I made? b. What is the worst part? c. What is the best part? d. How can it be improved? 4. Resetting goals

(continued)

Table 9.4 (Continued)

Week	Objective
Week 11 *Yeah!*	1. Weekly weigh-in 2. Checking in: diet, television, and physical activity logs. Plot your progress 3. How do I continue when I am no longer doing this program? 4. Homework
Week 12 *Nearly there*	1. Weekly weigh-in 2. Checking in: diet, television, and physical activity logs. Plot your progress 3. Planning termination: supervise but do not assist in the weigh-in and checking in stages 4. Homework
Week 13 *On my way!*	1. Weekly weigh-in 2. Checking in: diet, television, and physical activity logs. Plot your progress 3. Working on termination: student-run session to discuss the importance of continued adherence to the program 4. Homework
Week 14 *I'm off!*	1. Weekly weigh-in 2. Checking in for the last time 3. Termination 4. Award

always been on the heavy side, but her weight gain had accelerated in the fourth grade. She weighed 160 pounds and was 5 feet 1 inch tall at the time of this referral.

Lisa lived with her parents, Mr. and Mrs. Longs, and her 10-year-old brother in a suburban neighborhood. Both of her parents had full-time jobs. Since Lisa and her brother were not allowed to play outside for safety reasons, they completed their homework and then watched television until their parents' return.

Establishing a Working Alliance

The focus of the initial sessions was to establish a working alliance with Lisa, her family, and the school. The problem of Lisa's obesity was viewed from a family-systemic model (Goetz & Caron, 1999), and a working alliance among the family, therapist, and child is fundamental for the success of this model (Raue, Castonguay, & Goldfried, 1993). The family, particularly parents, as the proponent of change is one of the most effective modalities of treating pediatric obesity (Golan, Weizman, Apter, & Fainaru, 1998).

Baseline psychosocial, anthropometric, and lifestyle data were collected in this phase. At the initial meeting with Lisa, the counselor discussed the referral, explored Lisa's perception of the problem, and enlisted her participation in the OMP. Given the lack of empirically based short-term individualized obesity management programs, the counselor chose to use the multipronged OMP, in view of the fact that Lisa needed behavioral and dietary modifications with family and school support to ensure her adherence to the program.

The American Academy of Pediatricians describes childhood obesity as the most frustrating childhood condition to treat (Barlow & Dietz, 1998). There is no unitary cause for obesity. However, there is consensual data to indicate that the combination of excess caloric intake combined with low levels of physical activity result in obesity (Bray, 1987). Thus, interventions for children should be aimed at dietary and behavioral modifications with increased physical activity (see Table 9.2). Higher rates of success in weight management programs are associated with supportive, interactive families demonstrating parental skills aimed at the child's development of responsibility and self-image (Epstein, 1996; Epstein, Koeske, Wing, & Valoski, 1986; Epstein, Myers, Raynor, & Saelens, 1998).

The Home–School Collaboration

Home–school collaboration was pivotal for the success of this intervention. A "town meeting" with Lisa's parents (see Week 1 in Table 9.4), Lisa, and the counselor was the next step. Lisa chose Ms. Halferty, her homeroom teacher, as her in-school support person. Ms. Halferty was also included in the planning and execution of this program. At this meeting, the psychosocial and health consequences of Lisa's body weight were explored. Educational materials on obesity management were presented to her parents. The importance of the home–school collaboration for the success of the program was expounded. The Longs agreed to participate in the OMP and signed a contract indicating their willingness to actively assist Lisa with this program. Lisa's mother agreed to be Lisa's "sponsor." The role of the sponsor was to provide supervision, helping Lisa to complete homework assignments and stay on task, and to provide supportive nurturance at home. The structure of the 14-week OMP was outlined, and the responsibilities of the parent/sponsor were explained.

Baseline psychosocial and anthropometric data was collected at the second meeting. Psychosocial baseline data was collected on Lisa to assess her psychosocial health. There is substantive evidence to indicate that the psychosocial cost of obesity increases with the severity (Erermis et al., 2004; Wadden, Foster, Brownell, & Finley, 1984). Anxiety-depression, aggressiveness, social problems, social withdrawal, and internalizing and externalizing behavior are some of the problems that have been reported by caregivers of obese individuals (Erermis et al., 2004).

The focus of this phase of the intervention was to assess Lisa's caloric intake and expenditure and to determine her eating and activity patterns. Collecting baseline data (Figure 9.1) allows both the practitioner and the family to review the family's diet and activity patterns to identify the areas of over- and underconsumption, ascertaining problem behaviors (Barlow and Dietz, 1998).

Television (Dietz & Gortmaker, 1985; Gortmaker et al., 1996) and computer/video games have been purported to be the major cause of sedentary living among children (DuRant, Baranowski, Johnson, & Thompson, 1994; Marshall, Biddle, Gorely, Cameron, & Murdey, 2004). In addition to the sedentary lifestyle, these activities have been found to increase overall calorie consumption (Coon & Tucker, 2002; Jeffery & French, 1998; Kelder, Perry, Klepp, & Lytle, 1994; Kotz & Story, 1994; Kraak & Pelletier, 1998) through both the systematic advertising and consumption of calorie-dense snacks during these activities.

Lisa's task for the week was to complete daily (1) physical activity, (2) food, and (3) television and computer/video game logs for the next week (see Figure 9.2). The accuracy of recall records is affected by the frequency at which the record is completed. Accuracy is higher if the recording occurs close to the event (Baxter & Thompson, 2002). There is a rapid decay in memory, with poor reliability in recall after 24 hours (Armstrong et al., 2000). To facilitate Lisa's recall, both her parent sponsor and teacher provided her with reminders to complete her record. A note was sent home to Mr. and Mrs. Long (see Figure 9.3) outlining the program for the week. As the sponsor, Mrs. Long's role was to ensure that Lisa filled in her daily logs (Figure 9.4). In addition to being reminded at home, her classroom teacher was asked to remind Lisa to complete the log at the beginning and the end of the day.

Treatment and Intervention Strategy

After baseline data had been collated, the counselor and Lisa set up both short-term and intermediate goals (see Table 9.5). The treatment and intervention phase of the OMP focused on:

1. Providing nutrition and physical activity education (weeks 3 to 10)
2. Developing mastery over diet and activity patterns
3. Establishing a working collaborative relationship between home and school

The treatment and intervention phase was composed of education and behavior modification components. Nutrition education was directed at making Lisa and her family more astute in their dietary choices. Reading and understanding food labels, serving sizes, and nutrient content of foods were part of the nutrition education program. The aim was to increase the consumption of high-fiber foods and fruits and vegetables and decrease simple sugar and fat consumption. This behavioral modification program was aimed at making good food choices rather than caloric restriction. This type of intervention focuses on small behavior modifications that include eating at the same place, limiting

Lisa Long's Goal Chart Date: July 10, 2004

Date of Birth: 7–21–2004   Age: 11 years and 11 months

Height: 5 feet 1 inch (61 inches)   Weight: 160 pounds

BMI (kg/m²)

= weight in pounds * 0.455/height in inches * 0.025 * height in inches * 0.025

= (160 lbs) * 0.445/(61 inches * 0.025) * (61 inches * 0.025)

= 31.30 kg/m²

Goals:

   1. Diet

      Improve my eating habits so that I lose weight

      Stop snacking on cookies and candy

      Stop eating doughnuts

   2. Physical Activity:

      Start walking to school

      Walk around more when I am doing nothing

   3. Television:

      Watch only 2 hours of TV each day

My ideal BMI is 24.

Figure 9.1. Example of Lisa Long's Baseline Data and Goal Chart.

Name: Date: Day:

Program	Time		
	Started	Ended	

	Time
Breakfast:	
Lunch:	
Dinner (e.g., 2 slices of pizza and Coke):	
Snacks (e.g., a bag of potato chips):	

Activity	Time of Day	How long

Figure 9.2. Individual Food, Television, and Activity Logs.

Dear parent/guardian/sponsor, we are finally on our way.

This week Lisa will be collecting baseline data on

* The types of food that she eats,
* her physical activity patterns, and
* the television programs she watches and computer and video games that she plays each day.

Lisa has been advised to complete the logs over the course of the day. Please remind her to complete the log at least once a day.

After we have collected this information, we will better equipped to help Lisa attain her goal.

Thank you so much for helping Lisa with this program.

Sincerely,

Counselor

Figure 9.3. Example of Note to Parents.

food eaten to one or two helpings, and learning to substitute low-fat and no-fat products for full-fat products. Similarly, changes in physical activity are aimed at increasing lifestyle physical activity rather than implementing a structured physical activity program. Given the low maintenance costs, lifestyle physical activity changes (e.g., walking, playing games, household chores) are more likely to have enduring results (Kohl & Hobbs, 1998) compared to structured physical activity programs. Parental encouragement and support was espoused, and rewarding goal attainment was advocated. Recommended rewards included earning things that Lisa really wanted (e.g., providing her with the opportunity to gradually earn a new pair of shoes), choosing the family activity on family game night, or planning a family outing. Using food as an incentive was strongly discouraged. During this phase, both Lisa and her family learned alternative ways to eat without sacrificing palatability of foods. The decreased emphasis on television viewing had also given the family an opportunity to have more meaningful interactions with each other.

Baseline—Week 1: TV Viewing Log
Name: Lisa   Date: 15 July   Day: Thursday

Program	Time		
	Started	Ended	
Zoom	4:30 pm	5 pm	* *(30 minutes)*
Rugrats	5 pm	5:28 pm	* *(28 minutes)*
Simpsons	6 pm	6:30 pm	* *(30 minutes)*
Computer games	7 pm	9 pm	* *(120 minutes)*

* *Total amount of time spent watching television per day: 208 minutes (3 hours and 28 minutes)*

Food Log
Name: Lisa   Date: 15 July   Day: Thursday

	Time	Snacks	Time
Breakfast: 1 cup of dry Frosted Flakes with a cup of 2% milk, banana, small glass of orange juice, Pop Tart, a glass of milk	8 am	Chectos, soda	10:00 am
Lunch: 2 slices of pepperoni pizza, soda, 1 brownie	12:30 pm	Ice cream sandwich, potato chips	3 pm
Dinner: Quarter-pound burger, large fries, large soda	7 pm	Chocolate cake and chocolate milk	9 pm

Physical Activity Log
Name: Lisa   Date: 15 July   Day: Thursday

Activity	Time of day	How long
Played basketball in PE	12 pm	40 minutes
Walked home from the bus stop	4:15 pm	10 minutes

* *Total time spent on moderate to vigorous physical activity per day: 50 minutes*
* *All italicized information was completed by the counselor*

Figure 9.4. Example of Television, Food, and Activity Logs.

Table 9.5 Short-Term and Intermediate Goals

	Goal	Objectives
Television	Decrease fat- and sugar-dense snacks	Increase the consumption of good foods (green and yellow from the stoplight diet). Stop eating while watching TV. Measuring portions of food before eating them.
	Increase activity level during television viewing	Decrease the amount of time spent just sitting during a television program. Increase physical activity during commercial breaks. Increase the intensity of the physical activity so that metabolism is elevated.
	Limit the total time spent watching TV and playing computer and video games to 2 hours a day with the optimal goal being 1 hour a day	Plan television and computer time at the beginning of the week. Plan and have a list of alternate activities to fill in the "free" time. Plan and carry out a "turn your television off week."
Physical activity	Increase lifestyle physical activity and just keep on moving	Increase daily walking. Schedule a "walk to school" or "walk back from school day." Start walking with training buddy (mom). Find a physical activity or sport that I enjoy and increase participation in this activity. Join a club at school.
Diet	Increase good foods	Adopt and follow the 5-a-day plan. Decrease simple-carbohydrate consumption. Follow the food pyramid diet.
	Decrease soda consumption	Increase water intake; reduce or eliminate soda consumption.

Termination

The final phase (weeks 12 to 14) of the intervention was to provide both Lisa and her family with the tools to continue with the OMP after termination of the program. By this stage Lisa and her family had begun to employ behavioral modifications that resulted in better nutrition and physical activity choices. The increased involvement of the family in this program resulted in a renewed closeness, and the Long family was spending more time on family activities and outings. The termination process was directed toward empowering Lisa and her family to continue with positive physical activity and nutrition behaviors after the removal of active school support. By the end of the 14 weeks, Lisa had become more physically active and felt empowered to control her weight. This new confidence was also seen in her relationships with her peers. Lisa had not attained her goal BMI by the end of the program and decided that checking in with the counselor once a month for the rest of the academic year would provide adequate guidance for her to remain on the program.

Tools

Useful Web Sites and Additional Resources

Carter, J., Wiecha, J., Peterson, K., & Gortmaker, S. (2001). *Planet health: An interdisciplinary curriculum for teaching middle school nutrition and physical activity.* Champaign, IL: Human Kinetics.

CATCH. (2003). Coordinated approach to child health. Retrieved 13 July 2004 from http://www.catchinfo.org/

Cheung, L., Gortmaker, S., & Dart, H. (2001). *Eat well & keep moving: An interdisciplinary curriculum for teaching upper elementary school nutrition and physical activity.* Champaign, IL: Human Kinetics.

Epstein, L. H., & Squires, S. (1988). *The stoplight diet for children: An eight-week program for parents and children.* Boston: Little Brown and Company.

National Center for Chronic Disease Prevention and Health Promotion. (2004, 23 June). US obesity trends 1985 to 2002. Retrieved July 5, 2004, from http://www.cdc.gov/nccdphp/dnpa/obesity/trend/maps/index.htm

National Institute on Media and the Family. (2004). Fact sheet: Media use and obesity among children. Retrieved July 7, 2004, from http://www.mediafamily.org/facts/facts_tvandobchild_print.html

National Institutes of Health, National Heart, Lung, and Blood Institute. (1998). Clinical guidelines on the identification, evaluation, and treatment of overweight and obesity in adults—the evidence report. Obesity Research 6(S2):51S-209S [Published erratum appears in Obesity Research 6:464]. Retrieved July 2004 from http://www.nhlbi.nih.gov/guidelines/obesity/ob_home.htm

Rimm, S. (2004). *Rescuing the emotional lives of overweight children: What our kids go though—and how we can help.* Emmaus, PA: Rodale.

TV Turnoff Network. (2004, June 3). TV turnoff week. Retrieved June 14, 2004, from http://www.tvturnoff.org/index.htm

Weight Control Groups for Children

Childobesity.com

Shapedown.com/page2.htm

slimkids.com

thepathway.org

Nutrition: National Cancer Institute 5-a-Day Program

www.5aday.gov

Exercise

nutriteen.com

www.shapeup.org

Key Points to Remember

Some of the key points from this chapter are:

- Changing the dietary patterns of an obese child or adolescent requires a family-based initiative.
- A healthy diet can be fostered by
  - reducing the intake of dietary fat
  - reducing soda consumption
  - increasing dietary fiber
  - increasing fruit and vegetable consumption to five a day.
- Changes in lifestyle physical activity are more enduring than a structured physical activity program.
- Limiting television and computer viewing time increases the amount of time that is available for more meaningful engagement in lifestyle physical activities.
- Children are better able to lose weight and maintain their weight loss compared to adults.
- The key to a successful program is making enduring lifestyle changes.
- A paced program that spans a longer period is more effective in establishing enduring lifestyle changes.
- A collaborative family and school approach is more effective than either a family or a school program.

10

Design and Utility of Life Skills Groups in Schools

David R. Dupper

Getting Started

This chapter discusses the use of social skills training (SST) groups as a preventive or remedial intervention with children and youth. It begins with a discussion of social competence as a significant developmental accomplishment of children and youth who are experiencing problems. It discusses definitional problems surrounding the concept of social skills, best practices in the assessment of social skills, and research findings on the effectiveness of school-based SST groups as a promising intervention method for developing the social competencies of children and youth. This chapter then provides a brief discussion of issues related to cultural and racial differences and issues related to gender differences that should be considered in implementing SST interventions. Following this is an illustration of actions taken by a program staff in an effort to obtain support for and commitment to a social competence group in an elementary school. This chapter concludes with a summary of major points and additional resources.

What We Know

Social Competence as an Essential Aspect of Healthy Development

The development of social competence is an essential aspect of healthy normal development (LeCroy, 2002). Social competence is demonstrated through behaviors that parents, teachers, and peers consider important, adaptive, and functional in relation to environmental demands and age-appropriate societal expectations, such as peer acceptance and friendships, teacher and parental acceptance, and school adjustment (Gresham, Sugai, & Horner, 2001). According to Gresham (2002), "[T]he ability to interact successfully with peers and significant adults is one of the most important developmental accomplishments of children and youth" (p. 1029). Without such skills and competence, children and youth are more likely to experience friendship difficulties, inappropriately expressed emotions, and an inability to resist peer pressure (LeCroy, 1992). Clearly, the development of social competence should be considered an important developmental goal for all children (Katz, McClellan, Fuller, & Walz, 1995).

Unfortunately, substantial numbers of young people today lack the social competencies that protect against high-risk behaviors (Weissberg, Kumpfer, & Seligman, 2003). According to data from the Youth Risk Behavior Surveillance System (YRBSS), in 2003, 30.2% of high school students had ridden with a driver who had been drinking alcohol, 17.1% had carried a weapon, 33% had been in a physical fight; 8.5% had attempted suicide, 46.7% had had sexual intercourse, and 37% of sexually active students had not used a condom during their last sexual intercourse (Centers for Disease Control and Prevention, 2004). Moreover, the negative consequences of low levels of social competence in adolescents tend to persist into their adult years (Rose, 1998). Substantial research indicates that a lack of social skills in dealing with peers can lead to later maladjustments such as delinquency, dropping out of school, low academic achievement, antisocial behavior, alcoholism, and adult psychoses (Lope & Edelbaum, 1999).

The acquisition of social skills and the development of social competency are particularly important for students who demonstrate significant delays in cognitive, academic, and emotional/behavioral functioning and who meet the criteria specified in the Individuals With Disabilities Education Improvement Act (IDEA) for specific learning disabilities, mental retardation, emotional disturbance, and attention-deficit/hyperactivity disorder (Gresham & MacMillan, 1997).

Definitional Problems

Due to its relative simplicity as a construct and the fact that a very broad group of professional disciplines (e.g., social work, education, psychology, psychiatric nursing) have interest in it as a construct, "social skills is among the most widely misunderstood and ill-defined of all psychological constructs" (Merrell & Gimpel, 1998, p. 3). Gresham (1986) has divided the various definitions of social skills into three general categories: behavioral definitions, peer-acceptance definitions, and social validity definitions. The vast majority of studies have used behavioral definitions of social skills and defined them as "situation-specific behaviors that maximize the chances of reinforcement and minimize the chances of punishment based on one's social behavior" (Merrell & Gimpel, 1998, p. 5). Gresham, Sugai, and Horner (2001) defined social skills as "specific behaviors that an individual uses to perform competently or successfully on particular social tasks (e.g., starting a conversation, giving a compliment, entering an ongoing play group)" (p. 333). Peer-acceptance definitions of social skills depend upon popularity indices in defining social skills. For example, a child is viewed as being socially skilled if she is liked and accepted by her peers (Merrell & Gimpel, 1998). According to Gresham (1986), the social validity definition of social skills is a hybrid of these two categories and has received increasing empirical support since the 1980s. Based upon their extensive review of more than two decades of research, Caldarella and Merrell (1997) have developed an empirically based taxonomy of positive child and adolescent social skills. The five most common social skills dimensions identified through their meta-analysis are peer relations skills (e.g., compliments/praises/applauds peers), self-management skills (e.g., remains calm when problems arise, receives criticism well), academic skills (e.g., accomplishes tasks/assignments independently, listens to and carries out teacher's directions), compliance skills (e.g., follows rules, shares materials), and assertion skills (e.g., initiates conversations with others, questions unfair rules).

Assessment of Social Skills: Best Practices

The assessment process is an essential link between identifying children and adolescents with social skills deficits and developing an appropriate intervention plan (Merrell & Gimpel, 1998). The most direct and objective method of assessing social skills is through *direct observation*. All observational coding systems can be broken down into four general types of procedures: event recording, interval recording, time-sample recording, and duration and latency recording (Merrell & Gimpel, 1998). Space limitations will not allow for a detailed description of each of these general types. Therefore, readers seeking a detailed explanation of these coding systems should see Merrell and Gimpel (1998, pp. 63–69).

A second method that is widely used in assessing social skills in children and adolescents is *behavior rating scales*. Some widely used standardized behavior rating scales are the Behavioral Assessment System for Children (BASC; Reynolds & Kamphaus, 1992), the Social Skills Rating System (SSRS; Gresham & Elliott, 1990), the Preschool and Kindergarten Behavior Scales (PKBS; Merrell, 1994), and the Walker-McConnell Scales of Social Competence and School Adjustment (SSCSA; Walker & McConnell, 1995).

A third method used to assess social skills in children and adolescents is *sociometric techniques*. Rather than obtaining assessment data from teachers or outside observers, the defining feature of sociometric techniques is that data are obtained that assess the child's social status based on that child's peer group, usually within a classroom setting (Merrell & Gimpel, 1998). Sociometric methods usually "involve negative ranking or nomination procedures, or the use of negative characteristics to single out peers" (Merrell & Gimpel, 1998, p. 89) and can be divided into four general categories: peer nomination, picture sociometrics, "guess who" measures, and class play. See Merrell and Gimpel (1998) for a detailed description of these four sociometric techniques.

A fourth and final method of assessing social skills in children and adolescents is through *self-reports*. Through self-reports, objective data are obtained directly from the child or adolescent rather than from observers, teachers, or peers (Merrell & Gimpel, 1998). Self-report data are obtained through interviews and self-report tests, such as the Assessment of Interpersonal Relations (AIR; Bracken, 1993).

Research on the Effectiveness of Social Skills Training: Best Practices

Once an adequate assessment is completed, interventions that target specific social deficits can be implemented. One promising intervention method in developing social competencies of children and youth is SST. SST has been shown to be "perhaps the most promising new treatment model" for children and adolescents who are aggressive, disruptive, difficult to get along with, extremely shy or quiet, or unwilling to participate or socialize (LeCroy, 2002, p. 411). Rather than focusing solely on the elimination of problem behaviors, the primary focus of SST is the teaching of prosocial responses in situations that tend to elicit antisocial responses (LeCroy, 1983, 1992). Weissberg, Barton, and Shriver (1997) found that social competence promotion programs have had positive effects on adolescents' problem-solving skills, social relations with peers, school adjustment, and reductions in high-risk behaviors. Table 10.1 contains a listing of program components and best practices shown to be associated with positive program outcomes. Readers are encouraged to incorporate these components and best practices as much as possible in developing SST programs in school settings.

A number of programs have incorporated these essential components and have been found to be effective in enhancing social competencies in children and youth. See Table 10.2 for a brief description of these model or exemplary programs as well as for details on how to obtain more information about each program.

There is one important caveat. While SST shows great promise as an effective preventive intervention with many children and adolescents experiencing problematic behaviors, current research findings suggest that SST is not as beneficial for students classified into one of the high-incidence disability groups. This is particularly important, "given the documented social competence deficits of students with high-incidence disabilities" (e.g., specific learning disabilities, mental retardation, emotional disturbance, or attention-deficit/hyperactivity disorder) (Gresham, Sugai, & Horner, 2001, p. 335). Based on their meta-analysis of the relevant literature, Gresham, Sugai, and Horner (2001) suggest that SST "has not produced large, socially important, long-term, or generalized changes in social competence of students with high-incidence disabilities" (p. 331). These authors recommend that SST involving students with high-incidence disabilities should be more frequent and intense (because 30 hours of instruction spread over 10–12 weeks is not enough) and that SST must be "directly linked to the individual's social deficits....treatment cannot disregard the types of social skills deficits that the individual is displaying" (p. 341). They also go on to conclude that behaviors that lead to more powerful and immediate reinforcers will be performed more frequently than alternative behaviors. It is, therefore, critically important that the group leader ensures that the newly acquired social skills are

Table 10.1 Essential Components of Social Skills Training Programs: Best Practices

- Include a-n affective component (e.g., stress management)
- Include a cognitive component (e.g., problem solving)
- Include a behavioral component (e.g., social skills training)
- Include diverse and interactive teaching methods such as *modeling*, the process of learning a behavior by observing another person in the group perform that behavior; *role playing* or *behavioral rehearsal*, in which group members are asked to "try on" new modes of verbal and nonverbal behavior; *feedback*, in which following a role play, group members receive feedback from the group leader and group members about their performance; and *prompting* or *coaching*, when the group leader, prior to or during a role-play performance, provides verbal instructions to teach new social skills (each broad skill must be broken into its component parts so that it can be learned more easily)
- Focus on the selection of goals that group members will work on during the SST group
- Include behavioral homework assignments where group members are encouraged to practice newly acquired skills in their natural environment
- Incorporate generalization from the beginning of any SST program
- Be multiyear and allow children and youth to build on previous learning programs
- Emphasize a real-world application of skills to promote the generalization of skills
- Be implemented as early as possible in a child's life—ideally the training should begin in primary grades and continue through high school
- Focus on teaching children and youth to recognize and manage their emotions, appreciate the perspectives of others, establish positive goals, make good decisions, handle interpersonal situations and conflicts, and develop responsible and respectful attitudes and values about self, others, work, health, and community service

Sources: Caplan & Weissberg (1988); Gresham (2002); LeCroy (1983, 2002); Poland, Pitcher, & Lazarus (2002); Scott (n.d.); Weissberg, Kumpfer, & Seligman (2003).

reinforced more powerfully and immediately in the classroom and in the home than the older, problematic, competing behaviors.

What We Can Do

Groups are a natural context for social skills training. Groups allow for extensive use of modeling, support, feedback, and ongoing interaction with peers—all critical components of a successful SST (LeCroy, 2002). Moreover, groups are one of the most efficacious and cost-effective interventions in school settings (Krieg, Simpson, Stanley, & Snider, 2002).

Table 10.2 Model School-Based Programs Designed to Enhance Social Competence

Life Skills Training (LST) has been recognized as 1 of 10 model blueprint programs that have met the rigorous scientific standards established by the Center for the Study and Prevention of Violence at the University of Colorado at Boulder (Botvin, Mihalic, & Grotpeter, 1998). LST has also been recognized as a program that works by the Centers for Disease Control and Prevention, the American Medical Association, and the American Psychological Association. Detailed information about the *Life Skills Training program* can be found at http://www. lifeskillstraining.com

Promoting Alternative THinking Strategies (PATHS) has been recognized as 1 of 10 model blueprint programs that have met the rigorous scientific standards established by the Center for the Study and Prevention of Violence at the University of Colorado at Boulder (Greenberg, Kusche, & Mihalic, 1998). Detailed information about the PATHS program can be found at http://www. colorado.edu/cspv/blueprints/model/programs/PATHS.html

Second Step has been recognized as a model program by the Substance Abuse and Mental Health Services Administration, U.S. Department of Health and Human Services, and as an exemplary program by the U.S. Department of Education. Additional information about *Second Step* can be found at http://www. cfchildren.org/program_ss.shtml

The *School Survival Group* is designed for middle/junior high school students with school behavior problems. Findings from two studies (Dupper, 1998; Dupper & Krishef, 1993) have supported the short-term effectiveness of the School Survival Group. Hoagwood and Ervin (1997) in their review of school-based mental health services for children spanning a 10-year period found that only 16 out of 228 studies met the rigorous criteria of randomized assignment, inclusion of a control group, and use of standardized outcome measures and cited Dupper and Krishef as 1 of the 16 studies that met these three criteria. The curriculum for the School Survival Group can be found in the appendix of Dupper (2003)

The *Social Skills GRoup INtervention* (S.S. GRIN) is a generic social skills group intervention that combines social learning and cognitive-behavioral techniques. Since this group intervention was found to be equally effective across all of the subtypes of peer problems targeted, this study highlights the "potential value of utilizing generic social skills training protocols" (DeRosier, 2004, p. 196)

Although a number of authors (Elliott & Gresham, 1991; Merrell & Gimpel, 1998) have discussed models and guidelines for the teaching of social skills to children and adolescents in a small-group setting, the series of sequential steps outlined by LeCroy and Wooten (2002) is presented here due to its clarity and directness. The guidelines developed by LeCroy and Wooten (2002) can be useful to school social work practitioners interested in designing any SST program for children and adolescents in small-group settings:

1. Present the social skill being taught (e.g., solicit an explanation of the skill and get group members to provide a rationale for the skill).
2. Discuss the social skill (e.g., list the skill steps and get group members to give examples of using the skill).
3. Present a problem situation and model the skill (e.g., evaluate the performance and get group members to discuss the model).
4. Set the stage for role playing the skill (e.g., select the group members for role playing and get group members to observe the role play).
5. Have group members rehearse the skill (e.g., provide coaching if necessary and get group members to provide feedback on both verbal and nonverbal elements of role play).
6. Practice using complex skill situations (e.g., teach problem-solving skills and get group members to discuss situations and provide feedback).
7. Train for generalization and maintenance (e.g., encourage practice of skills outside the group and get group members to bring in their problem situations).

A description of one session from the School Survival Group, which incorporates many of these guidelines, can be found in Box 10.1. The entire curriculum for the School Survival Group can be found in the appendix of Dupper (2003). Readers should also see *Handbook of Child and Adolescent Treatment Manuals*, edited by Craig Winston LeCroy. In Chapter 5 of the book, LeCroy provides an overview of SST as well as a detailed description of each of the 11 group sessions of a social skills training group.

Issues Related to Cultural and Racial Differences

Cultural and racial differences must be considered in interpreting scores from standardized behavior rating scales and in developing SST programs. Cartledge (1996) discusses the teaching of social skills from a perspective of cultural diversity. In her book, she emphasizes the relationship between culture and social behavior and highlights the importance of ethnic identity relative to psychological adjustment and adaptive behavior. Cartledge argues that European- and American-based social skill assessments may not adequately reflect the social competence of culturally different students and that students' behaviors must

Box 10.1. Description of One Session From the School Survival Group

Session Two (Five Goals to Adolescent Behavior)
The leader begins by reviewing the five group rules. The leader next asks each group member to share the best thing that happened to them *in school* since the last group session. The leader begins by sharing something positive that happened to him/her, and other group members are encouraged to share. The leader states that each group session will begin by asking this question, and, therefore, group members are asked to make sure that at least one good thing happens to them in school so that they will have something to share at the beginning of each group.

The leader next asks the question: "Why do some students have difficulty getting along with teachers and other authority figures in school? Today, we are going to discuss the reason why we all behave in certain ways. All of us behave to meet certain needs that we have. What are some of these basic needs, beyond food, shelter, and clothing?"

"The first need we all have is to get *attention*. Why do we need attention? How does it feel when someone pays attention to us? We all need attention because we know we exist if someone is paying attention to us. If no one ever notices us, no matter what we do, we begin to feel like we don't exist. We all need attention, but some of us don't know how to get it in a positive way and *negative attention is better than no attention at all*. Unfortunately, some of us have only learned how to get negative attention (e.g., being the 'class clown,' being hyperactive, bizarre dress) rather than positive attention. Later in this group we will discuss ways to get positive attention rather than negative attention."

"The second need we all have is the need for *power*. We need to feel like we have a say in what happens to us. Unfortunately, many of you do not have much of an opportunity to exert your power in school (or at home). At your age, adults are always telling you what to do and you have little or no say in things that happen to you. I believe that this need for power is behind most of the problems between teenagers and adults. The adults want power over teens and the teens fight back because they want power, also. One of the most important things to remember in this group is that *teens always lose in power struggles with adults.* For example, who loses if you tell off a teacher? Who loses if you make an obscene gesture at the assistant principal for discipline? Students always lose. You cannot give a teacher a disciplinary referral to your teacher for her misbehavior in class, but she can sure give you one. You cannot suspend the principal, but he can sure suspend you. One of the things we will discuss later in group is how to not lose when you are in a power struggle with an adult."

"The third need which motivates behavior is the desire for *revenge.* Teens who feel hurt by life will strike back at others in an attempt to get even. Some people may resort to violence and destructive behavior in their efforts to get revenge. Remember that people who act this way are hurting very deeply inside and revenge is the way they have learned to deal with their hurt feelings. During this group we will discuss more productive ways of dealing with hurt."

"The fourth need that motivates some of our behavior is the need *to be left alone.* Some of us intentionally quit easily or avoid trying to do something altogether for fear that we may fail. This fear of failing school may lead us to start skipping school and dropping out of school at the first opportunity. Our thought is that if we don't try, then teachers and parents will give up on us and leave us alone. One of the goals of this group is to help you have more confidence in yourself and what you are able to do to survive in school."

"The fifth need many of us have is the need for *excitement.* Many of us are turned off by routine and become bored easily. Many teens believe that school is sooooo boring! And the way we deal with our boredom is by daydreaming, skipping school, doing alcohol or drugs, or anything that provides excitement. I hope that this group will help you to problem-solve ways to beat the boredom and routine of school.

(continued)

Box 10.1. (Continued)

The leader asks if anyone has questions or comments on these needs, which motivate much of teenage misbehavior in school. The leader asks for group members to state which of these needs he/she is attempting to meet and what is the behavior that he/she engages in to meet this need at school. The leader will then ask group members to discuss the consequences of each action if a student is "caught in the act" during the school day. The leader needs to stress that having attention and power, dealing with hurt, having more self-confidence, and having more excitement are worthwhile goals. What is essential is learning how to achieve these goals in ways that do not bring about negative consequences to us in school.

The leader concludes the group with each group member being asked to complete the following statement: "Today in group, I learned. ..."

be defined and interpreted within a cultural context. She cautions against interpreting culturally different behavior as social skills deficits or as pathological or dysfunctional. She states:

> Differences observed among racially and ethnically different groups of children may be more indicative of racial or ethnic differences than of deficits.... These behavioral patterns are rooted in the ways in which different groups are socialized. The issue with culturally different students, as with all students, is not to view these differences as pathological but to assess the degree to which they tend to support or interfere with success in later life. (Cartledge, 1996, p. 40)

Issues Related to Gender Differences

There are important differences between the sexes that must be taken into account in developing SST programs. For example, males tend to rate themselves higher than do females on measures of self-esteem in the areas of general academics, math, sports, and physical appearance (Stein, Newcomb, & Bentler, 1992). Cartledge (1996) states that, in comparison to males, "females appear to be more concerned with social relationships, more oriented toward a few close intimate relationships, more prone to avoid open conflict and express aggression in subtle exclusionary rather than physical ways, and more likely to use language to resolve conflicts" (Cartledge, 1996, p. 317). As a result of these differences, one important goal in developing SST groups is to focus on helping girls learn to behave assertively in a wider variety of situations, especially in those situations involving male participation (Cartledge, 1996). On a more macro level, Cartledge recommends that "[s]chool personnel need to examine more deliberately the way in which we socialize the sexes, taking pains to create cooperative environments and offer nonsexist curricula and literature in order to foster respect and adaptive behaviors between the sexes for the betterment of all" (1996, p. 344).

Tools and Practice Examples

Obtaining Support and Commitment: A Case Example

Prior to implementing a social skills group, it is important that the school social worker and mental health practitioner lay the necessary groundwork to ensure support and commitment to the program. The following excerpt from Rose (1998) is a good illustration of the actions taken by program staff in successfully implementing the autumn, winter, spring, and summer social competence group:

> After a series of discussions about children, classes, and teachers, the program staff and the school administrators agreed to implement a preventive social competence group work program in the third grade. The administrators indicated that several potential social competence difficulties seemed to be appearing among the third-grade children. They described incidents of quarreling in the cafeteria that were worrisome to them. The program staff and the school administrators were mature enough to grasp cognitive material presented in a preventive group. The principal discussed the ideas for a social competence development program with the three third-grade teachers who appeared amenable to a classroom approach.... The teacher's role included the coordination of program content with the rest of the curriculum, such as social studies and health education. The program content focused on increasing empathy, promoting a positive self-concept, and learning to analyze and apply problem-solving thinking skills in social situations involving peers. Prior to delivering the program, the leaders discussed the content and approach with the school staff who, after a brief delay, indicated their approval. The teacher provided the leaders with a class list.... All parents were informed of the program through a letter the teacher sent home. The leaders came one day to observe the class and to their surprise they saw several children acting aggressively toward their peers.... The class was divided into four smaller groups, each of which met in a corner of the classroom. Each group selected a member who chose a name of a season out of a hat.... The groups met once a week for 12 weeks...[The group members] played a board game the leaders had developed in which they each had to say what they felt in common school situations...[T]he members role played social situations and practiced responding in kindness to one another....In the middle phase, the members developed their assertiveness skills by practicing

making appropriate requests of peers…[T]here were many opportunities for role playing and modeling…[T]he members focused on social skills involved in making and keeping friends. They practiced initiating and maintaining conversations…[M]embers learned conflict identification and resolution skills and practiced using problem-solving thinking in stressful situations involving the aggressive actions of peers….The final phase emphasized consolidating gains, evaluating the group, and ending….Afterward, the teacher related the lessons learned to the over-all social studies curriculum, which was focused on the theme of people in the natural world. (pp. 119–122)

Resources

Skillstreaming the Elementary School Child: New Strategies and Perspectives for Teaching Prosocial Skills by Arnold P. Goldstein and Ellen McGinnis. Information about this program can be found at http://www.uscart.org/sselementary.htm

Skillstreaming the Adolescent: New Strategies and Perspectives for Teaching Prosocial Skills by Arnold P. Goldstein and Ellen McGinnis. Information about this program can be found at http://www.uscart.org/ssadolescent.htm

The Prepare Curriculum: Teaching Prosocial Competencies by Arnold P. Goldstein. *The Prepare Curriculum* presents a series of 10-course-length interventions grouped into three areas: reducing aggression, reducing stress, and reducing prejudice. Information about this program can be found at http://www.uscart.org/Prepare%20Curric.htm

An overview of the *Social Skills Training Program* by Goldstein and Pollock can be downloaded at http://www.users.globalnet.co.uk/~ebdstudy/strategy/socskils.htm.

The Overcoming Obstacles program includes a comprehensive relevant life skills curriculum taught as a stand-alone course and infused into other content areas. Information about this program can be found at http://www.overcomingobstacles.org

Key Points to Remember

- The development of social competence is an essential aspect of healthy normal development.
- Substantial numbers of young people today lack the social competencies that protect against high-risk behaviors.
- Social skills training (SST) has been shown to be the most promising new treatment model for children and adolescents who are aggressive, disruptive, difficult to get along with, extremely shy or quiet, or unwilling to participate or socialize.
- Social competence promotion programs have had positive effects on adolescents' problem-solving skills, social relations with peers, school adjustment, and reductions in high-risk behaviors.

- Social competence is best achieved by changing students' knowledge, skills, attitudes, beliefs, or behaviors by using interactive teaching techniques (e.g., role plays with peers) rather than lectures.
- SST should focus on youth during the critical middle-school/junior high years and consist of multiple years of intervention (e.g., "booster sessions") using a well-tested, standardized intervention with detailed lesson plans and student materials, delivered over extended periods, and continually reinforced in the school environment.
- Current research suggests that SST is not as beneficial for students classified into one of the high-incidence disability groups (e.g., specific learning disabilities, mental retardation, emotional disturbance, or attention-deficit/hyperactivity disorder). Consequently, it has been recommended that SST involving students with high-incidence disabilities should be more frequent and intense, and directly linked to the individual's social deficits, and the newly acquired social skills should be reinforced more powerfully and immediately in the classroom and in the home.
- It is important to include as many of the components and best practices, contained in Table 10.1, as possible in designing and implementing a SST program.
- European- and American-based social skills assessments may not adequately reflect the social competence of culturally different students.
- One important goal in developing SST groups is to focus on helping girls learn to behave assertively in a wider variety of situations, especially in those situations involving male participation.

References

Chapter I

Bangert-Drowns, R. L. (1988). The effects of school-based substance abuse education—A meta-analysis. *Journal of Drug Education, 18*, 243–264.

Best, J. A., Flay, B. R., Towson, S. M. J., Ryan, L. B., Perry, C., Brown, K. S., et al. (1984). Smoking prevention and the concept of risk. *Journal of Applied Social Psychology, 14*, 257–273.

Botvin, G. J. (1996). Substance abuse prevention through life skills training. In R. D. Peters & R. J. McMahon (Eds.), *Preventing childhood disorders, substance abuse, and delinquency.* Thousand Oaks, CA: Sage Publications.

Botvin, G. J., Baker, E., Botvin, E. M., Dusenbury, L., Cardwell, J., & Diaz, T. (1993). Factors promoting cigarette smoking among black youth: A causal modeling approach. *Addictive Behaviors, 18*, 397–405.

Botvin, G. J., Baker, E., Dusenbury, L., Tortu, S., & Botvin, E. M. (1990). Preventing adolescent drug abuse through a multimodal cognitive-behavioral approach: Results of a 3-year study. *Journal of Consulting and Clinical Psychology, 58*(4), 437–446.

Botvin, G. J., Baker, E., Renick, N., Filazzola, A. D., & Botvin, E. M. (1984). A cognitive-behavioral approach to substance abuse prevention. *Addictive Behaviors, 9*, 137–147.

Botvin, G. J., & Botvin, E. M. (1992). Adolescent tobacco, alcohol, and drug abuse: Prevention strategies, empirical findings, and assessment issues. *Developmental and Behavioral Pediatrics, 13*, 290–301.

Botvin, G. J., Dusenbury, L., Baker, E., & James-Ortiz, S. (1989). A skills training approach to smoking prevention among Hispanic youth. *Journal of Behavioral Medicine, 12*(3), 279–296.

Botvin, G. J., & Eng, A. (1982). The efficacy of a multicomponent approach to the prevention of cigarette smoking. *Preventive Medicine, 11*, 199–211.

Botvin, G. J., Eng, A., & Williams, C. L. (1980). Preventing the onset of cigarette smoking through life skills training. *Preventive Medicine, 9*, 135–143.

Botvin, G. J., Griffin, K. W., & Paul, E. (2003). Preventing tobacco and alcohol use among elementary school students through life skills training. *Journal of Child & Adolescent Substance Abuse, 12*(4), 1–17.

Botvin, G. J., Renick, N., & Baker, E. (1983). The effects of scheduling format and booster sessions on a broad spectrum psychosocial approach to smoking prevention. *Journal of Behavioral Medicine, 6*, 359–379.

Botvin, G. J., Schinke, S. P., Epstein, J. A., Diaz, T., & Botvin, E. M. (1995). Effectiveness of culturally focused and generic skills training approaches to alcohol and drug abuse prevention among minority adolescents: Two-year follow-up results. *Psychology of Addictive Behaviors, 9*(3), 183–194.

Bruvold, W. H. (1993). A meta-analysis of adolescent smoking prevention programs. *American Journal of Public Health, 83*(6), 872–880.

Bruvold, W. H., & Rundall, T. G. (1988). A meta-analysis and theoretical review of school based tobacco and alcohol intervention programs. *Psychology and Health, 2,* 53–78.

Burke, M. R. (2002). School-based substance abuse prevention: Political finger-pointing does not work. *Federal Probation, 66*(2), 66–72.

Caplan, M., Weissberg, R. P., & Grober, J. S. (1992). Social competence promotion with inner-city and suburban young adolescents: Effects on social adjustment and alcohol use. *Journal of Consulting & Clinical Psychology, 60*(1), 56–63.

Ennett, S. T., Tobler, N. S., Ringwalt, C. L., & Flewelling, R. L. (1994). How effective is drug abuse resistance education? A meta-analysis of Project DARE outcome evaluations. *American Journal of Public Health, 84*(9), 1394–1400.

Gottfredson, D. (1996). School-based crime prevention. In L. W. Sherman et al. (Eds.), *Preventing crime: What works, what doesn't, what's promising.* Report to the United States Congress, prepared for the National Institute of Justice.

Hops, H., Tildesley, E., & Lichtenstein, E. (1990). Parent–adolescent problem-solving interactions and drug use. *American Journal of Drug & Alcohol Abuse, 16*(3/4), 239–258.

Kinder, B., Pape, N., & Walfish, S. (1980). Drug and alcohol education programs: A review of outcome studies. *The International Journal of the Addictions, 15,* 1035–1054.

McAlister, A., Perry, C. L., Killen, J., Slinkard, L. A., & Maccoby, N. (1980). Pilot study of smoking, alcohol, and drug abuse prevention. *American Journal of Public Health, 70,* 719–721.

National Health Promotion Associates, Inc. (2002). Life Skills Training program. Retrieved July 12, 2004, http://www.lifeskillstraining.com

National Institute on Alcohol Abuse and Alcoholism. (2004). Statement by Ting-Kai Li, M.D. Fiscal Year 2005 President's Budget Request for the National Institute on Alcohol Abuse and Alcoholism. Bethesda, MD: U.S. Department of Health and Human Services. Retrieved July 26, 2004, http://www.niaaa.nih.gov/about/statement04.htm

Rosenbaum, D. P., & Hanson, G. S. (1998). Assessing the effects of school-based drug education: A six-year multilevel analysis of project D.A.R.E. *The Journal of Research in Crime and Delinquency, 35*(4), 381–412.

SAMHSA [Substance Abuse and Mental Health Services Administration]. (2004). *Results from the 2003 National Survey on Drug Use and Health: National Findings* (Office of Applied Studies, NSDUH Series H–25, DHHS Publication No. SMA 04–3964). Rockville, MD.

Schinke, S. P., Botvin, G. J., & Orlandi, M. A. (1991). *Substance abuse in children and adolescents.* Newbury Park, CA: Sage Publications.

Sherman, L. (2000). The safe and drug-free schools program. Brookings papers on education policy (pp. 125–171). Retrieved July 28, 2004, http://muse.jhu.edu/journals/brookings_papers_on_education_policy/v2000/2000.1sherman.html

Swisher, J. D., & Hoffman, A. (1975). Information: The irrelevant variable in drug education. In B. W. Corder, R. A. Smith, & J. D. Swisher (Eds.), *Drug abuse prevention: Perspectives and approaches for educators* (pp. 49–62). Dubuque, IA: William C. Brown.

Tobler, N. S. (1986). Meta-analysis of 143 adolescent drug prevention programs: Quantitative outcome results of program participants compared to a control group or comparison group. *Journal of Drug Issues, 16*(4), 537–567.

Tobler, N. S., & Stratton, H. H. (1997). Effectiveness of school-based drug prevention programs: A meta-analysis of the research. *Journal of Primary Prevention, 18*(1), 71–128.

White, D., & Pitts, M. (1998). Educating young people about drugs: A systematic review. *Addiction, 93*(10), 1475–1487.

Chapter 2

Alcoholism & Drug Abuse Weekly. (1999, April 19). Survey pinpoints substance use among elementary school students. *Alcoholism & Drug Abuse Weekly.*

American Academy of Pediatrics. (1998). Caring for your adolescent: Ages 12 to 21 (pamphlet).

Centers for Disease Control and Prevention. (2004). *Youth risk behavior surveillance: United States, 2003* (MMWR No. SS-2). Atlanta: U.S. Department of Health and Human Services.

DeMarsh, J. P., & Kumpfer, K. L. (1986). Family oriented interventions for the prevention of chemical dependency in children and adolescents. In S. Ezekoye, K. Kumpfer, & W. Bukoski (Eds.), *Childhood and chemical abuse: Prevention and early intervention* (pp. 117–152). New York: Haworth.

Erhard, R. (1999). Peer-led and adult-led programs—student perceptions. *Journal of Drug Education, 29*(4), 295–308.

Fisher, G. L., & Harrison, T. C. (2004). *Substance abuse: Information for school counselors, social workers, therapists, and counselors.* Boston: Pearson Education.

Flay, B. R., & Allred, C. G. (2003). Long-term effects of the Positive Action program. *American Journal of Health Behavior, 27* (Supp. 1), S6–S21.

Flay, B. R., Allred, C. G., & Ordway, N. (2001). Effects of the Positive Action program on achievement and discipline: Two matched-control comparisons. *Prevention Science, 2*(2), 71–89.

Gibson, R. L., Mitchell, M. H., & Basile, S. K. (1993). *Counseling in the elementary school: A comprehensive approach.* Boston: Allyn and Bacon.

Gonet, M. M. (1994). *Counseling the adolescent substance abuser: School-based intervention and prevention.* Thousand Oaks: CA: Sage.

Gottfredson, D. C., & Wilson, D. B. (2003). Characteristics of effective school-based substance abuse prevention. *Prevention Science, 4*(1), 27–38.

Griffin, K. W., Botvin, G. J., Nichols, T. R., & Doyle, M. M. (2003). Effectiveness of a universal drug abuse prevention approach for youth at high risk for substance use initiation. *Preventive Medicine, 36,* 1–7.

Hawkins, J. D., Catalano, R. F., Kosterman, R., Abbott, R., & Hill, K. G. (1999). Preventing adolescent health-risk behaviors by strengthening protection during childhood. *Archives of Pediatric and Adolescent Medicine, 153,* 226–234.

Hogan, J. A., Gabrielsen, K. R., Luna, N., & Grothaus, D. (2003). *Substance abuse prevention: The intersection of science and practice.* Boston: Allyn & Bacon.

Holleran, L. K., Kim, Y., & Dixon, K. (2004). Innovative approaches to risk assessment within alcohol prevention programming. In A. R. Roberts & K. R. Yeager

(Eds.), *Evidence-based practice manual: Research and outcome measures in health and human services* (pp. 677–684). New York: Oxford University Press.

Jenson, J. M. (1997). Risk and protective factors for alcohol and other drug use in childhood and adolescence. In M. W. Fraser (Ed.), *Risk and resilience in childhood* (pp. 117–139). Washington, DC: NASW Press.

Jenson, J. M., & Howard, M. O. (1991). Risk-focused drug and alcohol prevention: Implications for school-based prevention programs. *Social Work in Education, 13*(4), 246–256.

Knowles, C. R. (2001). *Prevention that works: A guide for developing school-based drug and violence prevention programs.* Thousand Oaks, CA: Corwin Press.

Kuhn, C., Swartzwelder, S., & Wilson, W. (1998). *Buzzed: The straight facts about the most used and abused drugs (from alcohol to ecstasy).* New York: W. W. Norton & Company.

Kumpfer, K. L. (2003). *Identification of drug abuse prevention programs: Literature review.* Retrieved July 13, 2004, from http://www.drugabuse.gov/about/organization/despr/hsr/da-pre/KumpferLitReview.html

Kumpfer, K. L., Alvarado, R., & Whiteside, H. O. (2003). Family-based interventions for substance use and misuse prevention. *Substance Use & Misuse, 38*(11–13), 1759–1787.

Lilja, J., Wilhelmsen, B. U., Larsson, S., & Hamilton, D. (2003). Evaluation of drug use prevention programs directed at adolescents. *Substance Use & Misuse, 38*(11–13), 1831–1863.

Marsiglia, F. F., Holleran, L., & Jackson, K. M. (2000). The impact of internal and external resources on school-based substance abuse prevention. *Social Work in Education, 22*(3), 145–161.

National Institute on Drug Abuse. (1997a). *Drug abuse prevention for at-risk groups* (NIH No. 97–4114). Rockville, MD: U.S. Department of Health and Human Services, National Institutes of Health.

National Institute on Drug Abuse. (1997b). *Drug abuse prevention: What works.* Rockville, MD: U.S. Department of Health and Human Services.

Pandina, R. J. (1996, September 19–20). *Risk and protective factor models in adolescent drug use: Putting them to work for prevention.* Paper presented at the National Conference on Drug Abuse Prevention Research: Presentations, papers, and recommendations, Washington, DC.

Parents' Resource Institute for Drug Education. (2003). *2002–03 PRIDE Surveys national summary for grades 4 thru 6.* Bowling Green, KY: Author.

Petosa, R. (1992). Developing a comprehensive health promotion program to prevent adolescent drug abuse. In G. W. Lawson & A. W. Lawson (Eds.), *Adolescent substance abuse: Etiology, treatment, and prevention* (pp. 431–450). Gaithersburg, MD: Aspen.

Rones, M., & Hoagwood, K. (2000). School-based mental health services: A research review. *Clinical Child and Family Psychology Review, 3*(4), 223–241.

St. Pierre, T. S., Mark, M. M., Kaltreider, D. L., & Campbell, B. (2001). Boys & girls clubs and school collaborations: A longitudinal study of a multicomponent substance abuse prevention program for high-risk elementary school children. *Journal of Community Psychology, 29*(2), 87–106.

Sarvela, P. D., Monge, E. A., Shannon, D. V., & Newrot, R. (1999). Age of first use of cigarettes among rural and small town elementary school children in Illinois. *Journal of School Health, 69*(10), 398–402.

Stoil, M. J., & Hill, G. (1996). *Preventing substance abuse: Interventions that work.* New York: Plenum.

Sullivan, T. N., & Farrell, A. D. (2002). Risk factors. In C. A. Essau (Ed.), *Substance abuse and dependence in adolescence: Epidemiology, risk factors and treatment* (pp. 87–118). New York: Taylor & Francis.

Sussman, S., Rohrbach, L. A., Ratel, R., & Holiday, K. (2003). A look at an interactive classroom-based drug abuse prevention program: Interactive contents and suggestions for research. *Journal of Drug Education, 33*(4), 355–368.

Tatchell, T. W., Waite, P. J., Tatchell, R. H., Durrant, L. H., & Bond, D. S. (2004). Substance abuse prevention in sixth grade: The effect of a prevention program on adolescents' risk and protective factors. *American Journal of Health Studies, 19*(1), 54–61.

Tobler, N. S. (1992). Drug prevention programs can work: Research findings. *Journal of Addictive Diseases, 11*(3), 1–28.

Wilson, D. B., Gottfredson, D. C., & Najaka, S. S. (2001). School-based prevention problem behaviors: A meta-analysis. *Journal of Quantitative Criminology, 17*(3), 247–272.

Chapter 3

Center for Disease Control and Prevention. (2004). *Youth risk behavior surveillance: United States, 2003* (MMWR No. SS-2). Atlanta: U.S. Department of Health and Human Services.

Dembo, R., Schmeidler, J., & Henly, G. (1996). Examination of the reliability of the Problem Oriented Screening Instrument for Teenagers (POSIT) among arrested youth entering a juvenile assessment center. *Substance Use & Misuse, 31*, 785–824.

Fisher, G. L., & Harrison, T. C. (2004). *Substance abuse: Information for school counselors, social workers, therapists, and counselors.* Boston: Pearson Education.

Gonet, M. M. (1994). *Counseling the adolescent substance abuser: School-based intervention and prevention.* Thousand Oaks, CA: Sage.

Havighurst, R. J. (1972). *Developmental tasks and education.* New York: David McKay.

Jeynes, W. (2002). The relationship between the consumption of various drugs by adolescents and their academic achievement. *American Journal of Drug Alcohol Abuse, 28*, 15–35.

Kirisci, L., Mezzich, A., & Tarter, R. (1995). Norms and sensitivity of the adolescent version of the Drug Use Screening Inventory. *Addictive Behaviors, 20*(2), 149–157.

Knight, J. R., Goodman, E., Pulerwitz, T., & DuRant, R. H. (2001). Reliability of the Problem Oriented Screening Instrument for Teenagers (POSIT) in adolescent medical practice. *Journal of Adolescent Health, 29*, 125–130.

Knight, J. R., Shrier, L. A., Bravender, T. D., Farrell, M., Bilt, J. V., & Shaffer, H. J. (1999). A new brief screen for adolescent substance abuse. *Archives Pediatrics & Adolescent Medicine, 153*, 591–596.

Martin, C. S., & Winters, K. C. (1998). Diagnosis and assessment of alcohol use disorders among adolescents. *Alcohol Health & Research World, 22*(2), 95–105.

Mayer, J., & Filstead, W. J. (1979). The Adolescent Alcohol Involvement Scale: An instrument for measuring adolescents' use and misuse of alcohol. *Journal of Studies on Alcohol, 40*, 291–300.

McLaney, M. A., & Boca, F. D. (1994). A validation of the Problem-Oriented Screening Instrument for Teenagers (POSIT). *Journal of Mental Health, 3*(3), 363–376.

McWhirter, J. J., McWhirter, B. T., McWhirter, E. H., & McWhirter, R. J. (2004). *At-risk youth: A comprehensive response.* Toronto, Canada: Brooks Cole.

Melchior, L. A., Rahdert, E., & Huba, G. J. (1994). *Reliability and validity evidence for the Problem Oriented Screening Instruments for Teenagers (POSIT).* Washington, DC: American Public Health Association.

Moberg, D. P., & Hahn, L. (1991). The Adolescent Drug Involvement Scale. *Journal of Adolescent Chemical Dependency, 2*(1), 75–88.

National Commission on Drug-Free Schools. (1990). *Toward a drug-free generation: A nation's responsibility.* Washington, DC: U.S. Government Printing Office.

Newcomb, M. D., & Bentler, P. M. (1989). Substance use and abuse among children and teenagers. *American Psychologist, 44*(2), 242–248.

Orenstein, A., Davis, R. B., & Wolfe, H. (1995). Comparing screening instruments. *Journal of Alcohol & Drug Education, 40*(3), 119–131.

Rahdert, E. R. (1991). *The Adolescent assessment/referral system manual.* Rockville, MD: U.S. Department of Health and Human Services, Alcohol, Drug Abuse, and Mental Health Administration.

Schwartz, R. H., & Wirtz, P. W. (1990). Potential substance abuse detection among adolescent patients: Using the Drug and Alcohol Problem (DAP) Quick Screen, a 30-item questionnaire. *Clinical Pediatrics, 29,* 38–43.

University of Michigan Institute for Social Research. (2003). Results from the 2003 Monitoring the Future Study. Retrieved July 25, 2004, from http://www.nida.nih.gov/Newsroom/03/2003MTFFactSheet.pdf

U.S. Department of Health and Human Services. (2000). *Healthy people 2010: Understanding and improving health* (2nd ed.). Washington, DC: U.S. Government Printing Office.

White, H. R., & Labouvie, E. W. (1989). Towards the assessment of adolescent problem drinking. *Journal of Studies on Alcohol, 50*(1), 30–37.

Winters, K. (1991). *Manual for the personal experience screening questionnaire (PESQ).* Los Angeles: Western Psychological Services.

Winters, K. C. (1992). Development of an adolescent alcohol and other drug abuse screening scale: Personal Experience Screening Questionnaire. *Addictive Behaviors, 17,* 479–490.

Winters, K. C. (2001a). Assessing adolescent substance use problems and other areas of functioning: State of the art. In P. M. Monti, S. M. Colby, & T. A. O'Leary (Eds.), *Adolescents, alcohol, and substance abuse: Reaching teens through brief interventions* (pp. 80–108). New York: Guilford.

Winters, K. C. (2001b). *Screening and assessing adolescents for substance use disorders (DHHS Publication No. SMA 01–3493).* Rockwall, MD: Center for Substance Abuse Treatment, U.S. Department of Health and Human Services.

Winters, K. C., Latimer, W. W., & Stinchfield, R. D. (1999). DSM-IV criteria for adolescent alcohol and cannabis use disorders. *Journal of Studies on Alcohol, 60,* 337–344.

Chapter 4

Alan Guttmacher Institute. (2002). Teenagers' sexual and reproductive health. *Facts in Brief, January, 2002.* New York: Alan Guttmacher Institute. Retrieved November 1, 2003, from http://www.agi-usa.org

Centers for Disease Control and Prevention. (2002). *Young people at risk: HIV/AIDS among America's youth.* Atlanta, GA: U.S. Department of Health and Human Services, Centers for Disease Control and Prevention. Retrieved December 18, 2004, from http://www.cdc.gov/hiv

Centers for Disease Control and Prevention. (2003a). *HIV/AIDS surveillance report: Cases of HIV infection and AIDS in the United States, 2003.* Atlanta, GA: U.S. Department of Health and Human Services, Centers for Disease Control and Prevention (pp. 1–9). Retrieved December 18, 2004, from http://www.cdc.gov/hiv/stats/hasrlink.htm

Centers for Disease Control and Prevention. (2003b). *Youth risk behavior surveillance 2003.* Atlanta, GA: U.S. Department of Health and Human Services, Centers for Disease Control and Prevention. Retrieved December 17, 2004, from www.cdc.gov.

Centers for Disease Control and Prevention. (2003c). *HIV strategic plan through 2005.* Atlanta, GA: U.S. Department of Health and Human Services, Centers for Disease Control and Prevention. Retrieved December 18, 2004, from http://www. cdc.gov/nchstp/od/hiv_plan/Table%20of%20Contents.htm

Collins, J., Robin, L., Wooley, S., Fenley, D., Hunt, P., Taylor, J., et al. (2002). Programs-that-work: CDC's guide to effective programs that reduce health-risk behavior of youth. *Journal of School Health, 72*(3), 93–99.

Coyle, K., Basen-Engquist, K., Kirby, D., Parcel, G., Banspach, S., Harrist, R., et al. (1999). Short term impact of Safer-Choices: A multi-component, school-based HIV, other STD, and pregnancy prevention program. *Journal of School Health, 69*(5), 181–188.

Fisher, J. D., Fisher, W. A., Bryan, A. D., & Misovich, S. J. (1998). Information-Motivation-Behavioral Skills Model based HIV risk behavior change intervention for inner city youth. *Health Psychology, 21*(2), 177–186.

Jemmott, J., Jemmott, L., & Fong, G. (1992). Reductions in HIV risk associated sexual behaviors among black male adolescents: Effects of an AIDS prevention program. *American Journal of Public Health, 82*(3), 372–377.

Jemmott, J. B., Jemmott, L. S., Fong, G. T., & McCaffree, K. (1998). Abstinence and safer sex: HIV risk-reduction interventions for African American adolescents. *Journal of the American Medical Association, 279*(19), 1529–1536.

Johnson, B. T., Carey, M. P., Marsh, K. L., Levin, K. D., & Scott-Sheldon, J. (2003). Interventions to reduce sexual risk for the Human Immunodeficiency Virus in adolescents, 1985–2000. *Archives of Pediatric and Adolescent Medicine, 157,* 381–388.

Kipke, M. D., Boyer, C., & Hein, K. (1993). An evaluation of an AIDS risk reduction education and skills training (ARREST) program. *Journal of Adolescent Health, 14*(7), 533–539.

Kirby, D. (1999). Reflections on two decades of research on teen sexual behavior and pregnancy. *Journal of School Health, 69*(3), 89–94.

Kirby, D. (2002). The impact of schools and school programs upon adolescent sexual behavior. *Journal of Sex Research, 39*(1), 27–33.

Kirby, D., Barth, R. P., Leland, N., & Fetro, J. V. (1991). Reducing the risk: Impact of a new curriculum on sexual risk-taking. *Family Planning Perspectives, 23*(6), 253–263.

Lohrmann, D. K., Blake, S., Collins, T., Windsor, R., & Parrillo, A. V. (2001). Evaluation of school-based HIV prevention education programs in New Jersey. *Journal of School Health, 71*(6), 207–211.

Main, D., Iverson, D., McGloin, J., Banspach, S. W., Collins, J. L., Rugg, D. L., et al. (1994). Preventing HIV infection among adolescents: Evaluation of a school-based education program. *Preventive Medicine, 23*(4), 409–417.

Misovich, S. J., Fisher, W. A., Fisher, J. D., Figueroa-Richmond, B., Bryan, A., & Muller, L. (2000). *Information–Motivation–Behavioral Skills HIV Prevention Program: Teacher's manual and natural opinion leader training manual.* Published by Films for the Humanities and Sciences (films.com). Retrieved December 11, 2004, from http://www.films.com/Films_Home/item.cfm?s=1&bin=8801

Remafedi, G. (1994). Cognitive and behavioral adaptations to HIV/AIDS among gay and bisexual adolescents. *Journal of Adolescent Health, 15,* 142–148.

Rotheram-Borus, M. J., Gwadz, M., Fernandez, M. I., & Srinivasan, S. (1998). Timing of HIV interventions on reductions in sexual risk among adolescents. *American Journal of Community Psychology, 26,* 73–96.

Rotheram-Borus, M. J., Kooperman, C., Haignere, C., & Davies, M. (1991). Reducing HIV sexual risk behaviors among runaway adolescents. *JAMA: Journal of the American Medical Association, 266,* 1237–1241.

Rotheram-Borus, M. J., Reid, H., & Rosario, M. (1994). Factors mediating changes in sexual HIV risk behaviors among gay and bisexual male adolescents. *American Journal of Public Health, 84*(12), 1938–1946.

Rotheram-Borus, M., Van Rossem, R., Gwadz, M., Koopman, C., & Lee, M. (1997). *Street smart.* Retrieved December 18, 2004, from http://chipts.ucla. edu/interventions/manuals/intervstreetsmart.html.

St. Lawrence, J., Brasfield, T., Jefferson, K., Alleyne, E., O'Brannon, R., & Shirley, A. (1995). A cognitive-behavioral intervention to reduce African-American adolescents' risk for HIV infection. *Journal of Consulting and Clinical Psychology, 63*(2), 221–237.

Stanton, B., Li, X., Ricardo, I., Galbraith, J., Feigelman, S., & Kaljee, L. A. (1996). A randomized, controlled effectiveness trial of an AIDS prevention program for low-income African-American youths. *Archives of Pediatric and Adolescent Medicine, 151*(4), 398–406.

Stryker, J., Samuels, S. E., & Smith, M. D. (1994). Condom availability in schools: The need for improved program evaluations. *American Journal of Public Health, 84*(12), 1901–1906.

Chapter 5

Centers for Disease Control and Prevention. (2003a). *Sexually transmitted disease surveillance, 2003: Adolescents and young adults.* Atlanta, GA: U.S. Department of Health and Human Services, September 2004. Retrieved on December 20, 2004, from http://www.cdc.gov/std/stats/adol.htm

Centers for Disease Control and Prevention. (2003b). *Youth risk behavior surveillance 2003.* Atlanta, GA: U.S. Department of Health and Human Services, Centers for Disease Control and Prevention. Retrieved December 17, 2004, from www.cdc.gov

Rotheram-Borus, M., Van Rossem, R., Gwadz, M., Koopman, C., & Lee, M. (1997) *Street smart.* Retrieved December 18, 2004, from http://chipts.ucla.edu/interventions/manuals/intervstreetsmart.html

Southwestern, University of Texas Southwestern Medical Center at Dallas (n.d.). *HIV prevention toolbox: Street smart*. Retrieved December 21, 2004, from http://www3.utsouthwestern.edu/preventiontoolbox/interven/streetsmart.htm

Chapter 6

Alderman, T. A. (1997). *The scarred soul: Understanding and ending self-inflicted violence*. Oakland, CA: New Harbinger Publications.

Allen, C. (1995). Helping with deliberate self-harm: Some practical guidelines. *Journal of Mental Health, 4*(3), 243–250.

Chitsabesan, P., Harrington, R., Harrington, V., & Tomenson, B. (2003). Predicting repeat self-harm in children: How accurate can we expect to be? *European Child & Adolescent Psychiatry, 12*, 23–29.

Derouin, A., & Bravender, T. (2004). Living on the edge: The current phenomenon of self-mutilation in adolescents. *American Journal of Maternal/Child Nursing, 29*(1), 12–18.

Evans, J. (2000). Interventions to reduce repetition of deliberate self-harm. *International Review of Psychiatry, 12*, 44–47.

Favazza, A. R. (1989). Why patients mutilate themselves. *Hospital and Community Psychiatry, 40*, 137–145.

Favazza, A. R. (1998). The coming of age of self-mutilation. *Journal of Nervous and Mental Disorders, 186*, 259–268.

Favazza, A. R. (1999). Self-mutilation. In D. G. Jacobs (Ed.), *The Harvard Medical School guide to suicide assessment and intervention* (pp. 125–145). San Francisco: Jossey Bass.

Favazza, A. R., & Conterio, K. (1988). The plight of chronic self-mutilators. *Community Mental Health Journal, 24*(1), 22–30.

Favazza, A. R., & Conterio, K. (1989). Female habitual self-mutilation. *Acta Psychiatrica Scandinavica, 79*, 283–289.

Favazza, A. R., DeRosear, L., & Conterio, K. (1989). Self-mutilation and eating disorders. *Suicide and Life-Threatening Behaviors, 19*, 352–361.

Favazza, A. R., & Rosenthal, R. (1990). Varieties of pathological self mutilation. *Behavioral Neurology, 3*, 77–85.

Favazza, A. R., & Simeon, D. (1995). Self-mutilation. In E. Hollander & D. J. Stein (Eds.), *Impulsivity and aggression* (pp. 185–200). Chicester, England: John Wiley and Sons.

Froeschle, J., & Moyer, M. (2004). Just cut it out: Legal and ethical challenges in counseling students who self-mutilate. *Professional School Counseling, 7*(4), 231.

Fryer, M. R. (1988). Suicide attempts in patients with borderline personality disorder. *American Journal of Psychiatry, 145*, 737–739.

Grossman, R., & Siever, L. (2001). Impulsive self-injurious behaviors: Phenomenology, neurobiology and treatment. In D. Simeon & E. Hollander (Eds.), *Self injurious behaviors* (pp. 117–148). Washington, DC: American Psychiatric Publishing.

Guertin, T., Lloyd-Richardson, E., Spirito, A., Donaldson, D., & Boergers, J. (2001). Self-mutilative behavior in adolescents who attempt suicide by overdose. *Journal of the American Academy of Child and Adolescent Psychiatry, 40*(9), 1062–1074.

Gunnell, D., & Frankel, S. (1994). Prevention of suicide: Aspirations and evidence. *British Medical Journal, 308*, 1227–1233.

Herpertz, S. (1995). Self-injurious behavior: Psychopathological and nosological characteristics in subtypes of self-injurers. *Acta Psychiatrica Scandinavica, 91,* 57–68.

Himber, J. (1994). Blood rituals, self-cutting in female psychiatric patients. *Psychotherapy, 31,* 620–631.

Ivanoff, A., Linehan, M. M., & Brown, M. (2001). Dialectic behavior therapy for impulsive self-injurious behaviors. In D. Simeon & E. Hollander (Eds.), *Self injurious behaviors: Assessment and treatment* (pp. 437–459). Washington, DC: American Psychiatric Publishing.

Kahan, J., & Pattison, E. M. (1984). Proposal for a distinctive diagnosis: The deliberate self-harm syndrome. *Suicide and Life-Threatening Behavior, 14,* 17–35.

Kreftman, N., & Casey, P. (1988). The repetition of parasuicide: An epidemiological and clinical study. *British Journal of Psychiatry, 153,* 792–800.

Kumar, G., Pepe, D., & Steer, R. A. (2004). Adolescent psychiatric inpatients' self reported reasons for cutting themselves. *Journal of Mental Diseases, 192*(12), 830–836.

Osuch, E. A., Noll, J. G., & Putnam, F. W. (1999). The motivation for self-injury in psychiatric inpatients. *Psychiatry, 62,* 334–345.

Pattison, E. M., & Kahan, J. (1983). The deliberate self-harm syndrome. *American Journal of Psychiatry, 140,* 867–872.

Pipher, M. (1994). *Reviving Ophelia: Saving the selves of adolescent girls.* New York: Ballentine Books.

Sandman, C. A., & Touchette, P. (2002). Opioids and the maintenance of self-injurious behavior (pp. 191–204). In S. R. Schroeder, M. L. Oster-Granite, & T. Thompson (Eds.), *Self-injurious behavior: Gene-brain-behavior relationships* (pp. 191–204). Washington, DC: American Psychological Association.

Simeon, D., & Favazza, A. R. (2001). Self-injurious behaviors: Phenomenology & assessment. In D. Simeon & E. Hollander (Eds.), *Self-injurious behaviors: Assessment and treatment* (pp. 1–28). Washington, DC: American Psychiatric Publishing.

Sonneborn, C. K., & Vanstraelen, P. M. (1992). A retrospective study of self-inflicted burns. *General Hospital Psychiatry, 13,* 404–407.

Suyemoto, K. (1998). The functions of self-mutilation. *Clinical Psychology Review, 18*(5), 531–554.

Taiminen, T. J., Kallio-Soukainen, K., Nokso-Koivisto, H., Kaljonen, A., & Helenuis, H. (1998). Contagion of deliberate self-harm among adolescent inpatients. *Journal of the American Academy of Child and Adolescent Psychiatry, 37*(2), 211–217.

van der Kolk, B. A., & Fisler, R. E. (1994). Child abuse and neglect and loss of self regulation. *Bulletin of the Menninger Clinic, 58,* 145–168.

van der Kolk, B. A., Perry, C. J., & Herman, J. L. (1991). Childhood origins of self-destructive behavior. *American Journal of Psychiatry, 148*(12), 1665–1671.

Walsh, B. W., & Rosen, P. M. (1988). *Self-mutilation: Theory, research and treatment.* New York: Guilford.

Yaryura-Tobias, J. A., Nezitoglu, F. A., & Kaplan, S. (1995). Self-mutilation, anorexia, and dysmenorrhea in obsessive-compulsive disorder. *International Journal of Eating Disorders, 17,* 33–38.

Zila, M. L., & Kiselica, M. S. (2001). Understanding and counseling self-mutilation in female adolescents and young adults. *Journal of Counseling and Development, 79,* 46–79.

Chapter 7

Anderson, H. (1997). *Conversation, language, and possibilities: A postmodern approach to therapy.* New York: Basic.
Anderson, H., & Goolishian, H. (1988). Human sys-tems as linguistic systems: Evolving ideas about the implications for theory and practice. *Family Process, 27,* 371–393.
Anthony, E. J. (1984). The St. Louis risk research project. In N. F. Watt, E. J. Anthony, L. C. Wynne, & J. Roth (Eds.), *Children at risk for schizophrenia: A longitudinal perspective* (pp. 105–148). Cambridge, UK: Cambridge University Press.
Bennett-Goleman, T. (2001). *Emotional alchemy: How the mind can heal the heart.* New York: Harmony.
Berg, I. K., & Miller, S. D. (1992). *Working with the problem drinker: A solution-focused approach.* New York: Norton.
Berg, I. K., & Steiner, T. (2003). *Children's solution work.* New York: Norton.
Conterio, K., & Lader, W. (1998). *Bodily harm: The breakthrough treatment program for self-injurers.* New York: Hyperion.
Czikszentmihalyi, M. (1997). *Finding flow.* New York: Basic.
De Shazer, S. (1988). *Clues: Investigating solutions in brief therapy.* New York: Norton.
De Shazer, S. (1991). *Putting difference to work.* New York: Norton.
Epston, D. (1998). *Catching up with David Epston: Collection of narrative-based papers 1991–1996.* Adelaide, South Australia: Dulwich Centre Publications.
Favazza, A. R. (1998). *Bodies under siege: Self-mutilation and body modification in culture and psychiatry* (2nd ed.). Baltimore, MD: Johns Hopkins University Press.
Favazza, A. R., & Selekman, M. (2003/April). *Self-injury in adolescents.* Annual Spring Conference of the Child and Adolescent Centre, London, Ontario, Canada.
Fredrickson, B. (2002). *Positive emotion.* In C. R. Snyder & S. J. Lopez (Eds.), Handbook of positive psychology (pp. 120–135). New York: Oxford University Press.
Hanh, T. N. (2001). *Anger.* New York: Riverhead.
Hanh, T. N. (2003). *Creating true peace: Ending violence in yourself, your family, your community, and the world.* New York: Free Press.
O'Hanlon, W. H. (1987). *Taproots: Underlying principles of Milton H. Erickson's therapy and hypnosis.* New York: Norton.
O'Hanlon, W. H., & Weiner-Davis, M. (1989). *In search of solutions: A new direction in psychotherapy.* New York: Norton.
Peterson, C., & Seligman, M. E. P. (2004). *Character strengths and virtues: Handbook and classification.* New York: Oxford University Press.
Santisteban, D. A., Muir, J. A., Mena, M. P., & Mitrani, V. B. (2003). Integrated borderline family therapy: Meeting the challenge of treating adolescents with borderline personality disorder. *Psychotherapy: Theory, Research, Practice, & Training, 40,* 251–264.
Schwartz, B. (2004). *The paradox of choice: Why more is less.* New York: HarperCollins.
Selekman, M. D. (1997). *Solution-focused therapy: Harnessing family strengths for systemic change.* New York: Guilford.
Selekman, M. D. (2005). *Pathways to change: Brief therapy solutions with difficult adolescents* (2nd ed.). New York: Guilford.
Selekman, M. D. (2006). *Working with self-harming adolescents. A collaborative, strengths-based therapy approach.* New York: Norton.

Seligman, M. E. P. (2002). *Authentic happiness.* New York: Free Press.
Seligman, M. E. P., Reivich, K., Jaycox, J., & Gillham, J. (1995). *The optimistic child.* New York: Houghton-Mifflin.
Taffel, R., & Blau, M. (2001). *The second family: How adolescent power is challenging the American family.* New York: St. Martin's.
White, M. (1995). *Re-authoring lives: Interviews & essays.* Adelaide, South Australia: Dulwich Centre Publications.
White, M., & Epston, D. (1990). *Narrative means to therapeutic ends.* New York: Norton

Chapter 8

Agras, W. S., & Apple, R. F. (1997). *Overcoming eating disorders: A cognitive-behavioral treatment for bulimia nervosa and binge eating disorder.* San Antonio, TX: Psychological Corporation.
Agras, W. S., & Apple, R. F. (2002). Understanding and treating eating disorders. In F. W. Kaslow & T. Patterson (Eds.), *Comprehensive handbook of psychotherapy: Vol. 2. Cognitive behavioral approaches* (pp. 189–212). New York: Wiley.
American Psychiatric Association. (2000). *Diagnostic and statistical manual of mental disorders* (4th ed., text revision). Washington, DC: Author.
Bowers, W. A., Evans, K., & Van Cleve, L. (1996). Treatment of adolescent eating disorders. In M. A. Reineke, F. M. Dattilio, & A. Freeman (Eds.), *Cognitive therapy with children and adolescents: A casebook for clinical practice* (pp. 227–250). New York: Guilford.
Eisler, I., Dare, C., Hodes, M., Russell, G., Dodge, E., & Le Grange, D. (2000). Family therapy for adolescent anorexia nervosa: The results of a controlled comparison of two family interventions. *Journal of Child Psychology and Psychiatry, 41,* 727–736.
Fairburn, C. G., Agras, W. S., & Wilson, G. T. (1992). The research on the treatment of bulimia nervosa: Practical and theoretical implications. In G. H. Anderson & S. H. Kennedy (Eds.), *The biology of feast and famine: Relevance to eating disorders* (pp. 318–340). New York: Academic.
Fairburn, C. G., Marcus, M. D., & Wilson, G. T. (1993). Cognitive-behavioral therapy for binge eating and bulimia nervosa: A comprehensive treatment manual. In C. G. Fairburn & G. T. Wilson (Eds.), *Binge eating: Nature, assessment, and treatment* (pp. 361–404). New York: Guilford.
Halmi, K. (2003). Eating disorders. In A. Martin, L. Scahill, D. Charney, & J. Leckman (Eds.), *Pediatric psychopharmacology* (pp. 592–602). New York: Oxford University Press.
Hoek, H. W., & van Hoeken, D. (2003). Review of the prevalence and incidence of eating disorders. *International Journal of Eating Disorders, 34,* 383–396.
Kotwal, R., McElroy, S., & Malhotra, S. (2003). What treatment data support Topiramate in bulimia nervosa and binge eating disorder? What is the drug's safety profile? How is it used in these conditions? *Eating Disorders, 11,* 71–75.
Lock, J., Le Grange, D., Agras, W. S., & Dare, C. (2001). *Treatment manual for anorexia nervosa: A family-based approach.* New York: Guilford.
Nicholls, D., & Bryant-Waugh, R. (2003). Children and young adolescents. In J. Treasure, U. Schmidt, & E. van Furth (Eds.), *Handbook of eating disorders* (pp. 415–433). New York: Wiley.

Schmidt, U. (1998). Eating disorders and obesity. In P. Graham (Ed.), *Cognitive-behaviour therapy for children and families* (pp. 262–281). Cambridge: Cambridge University Press.

Sim, L., Sadowski, C., Whiteside, S., & Wells, L. (2004). Family-based therapy for adolescents with anorexia nervosa. *Mayo Clinic Proceedings, 79*, 1305–1308.

Chapter 9

Armstrong, A. M., MacDonald, A., Booth, I. W., Platts, R. G., Knibb, R. C., & Booth, D. A. (2000). Errors in memory for dietary intake and their reduction. *Applied Cognitive Psychology, 14*(2), 183–192.

Barlow, S. E., & Dietz, W. H. (1998). Obesity evaluation and treatment: Expert committee recommendations. *Pediatrics, 102*(3), e29. Retrieved November 2004 from http://www.pediatrics.org/cgi/content/full/102/3/e29

Baxter, S. D., & Thompson, W. O. (2002). Accuracy by meal component of fourth-graders' school lunch recalls is less when obtained during a 24-hour recall than as a single meal. *Nutrition Research, 22*(6), 679–684.

Bellizzi, M. C., & Dietz, W. H. (1999). Workshop on childhood obesity: Summary of the discussion. *American Journal of Clinical Nutrition, 70*(1), 173S-5.

Bray, G. A. (1987). Obesity—a disease of nutrient or energy imbalance? *Nutrition Reviews, 45*, 33–43.

Brownell, K. D., Kelman, J. H., & Stunkard, A. J. (1983). Treatment of obese children with and without their mothers: Changes in weight and blood pressure. *Pediatrics, 71*(4), 515–523.

Buckley, M. A., & Zimmermann, S. H. (2003). *Mentoring children and adolescents: A guide to the issues.* Westport, CT: Praeger Publishers.

Carter, J., Wiecha, J., Peterson, K., & Gortmaker, S. (2001). *Planet health: An interdisciplinary curriculum for teaching middle school nutrition and physical activity.* Champaign, IL: Human Kinetics.

CATCH. (2003). *Coordinated approach to child health.* Retrieved July 13, 2004 from http://www.catchinfo.org/

Cheung, L., Gortmaker, S., & Dart, H. (2001). *Eat well & keep moving: An interdisciplinary curriculum for teaching upper elementary school nutrition and physical activity.* Champaign, IL: Human Kinetics.

Coates, T. J., Jeffery, R. W., Slinkard, L. A., Killen, J. D., & Danaher, B. G. (1982). Frequency of contact and monetary reward in weight loss, lipid change and blood pressure reduction with adolescents. *Behavior Therapy, 13*, 175–185.

Coon, K. A., & Tucker, K. L. (2002). Television and children's consumption patterns: A review of the literature. *Minerva Pediatrics, 54*, 423–436.

Dietz, W. (1991). Physical activity and childhood obesity. *Nutrition, 7*(4), 295–296.

Dietz, W. H., Jr., & Gortmaker, S. L. (1985). Do we fatten our children at the television set? Obesity and television viewing in children and adolescents. *Pediatrics, 75*(5), 807–812.

DuRant, R. H., Baranowski, T., Johnson, M., & Thompson, W. O. (1994). The relationship among television watching, physical activity and body composition of young children. *Pediatrics, 94*, 449–455.

Epstein, L. H. (1996). Family based behavioral intervention for obese children. *International Journal of Obesity, 20*, S14–S21.

Epstein, L. H., Koeske, R., Wing, R. R., & Valoski, A. (1986). The effects of family variables on child weight change. *Health Psychology, 5*, 1–11.

Epstein, L. H., Myers. M. D., Raynor, H. A., & Saelens, B. E. (1998). Treatment of pediatric obesity. *Pediatrics, 101*, 554–570.

Epstein, L. H., & Squires, S. (1988). *The stoplight diet for children: An eight-week program for parents and children.* Boston: Little Brown and Company.

Epstein, L. H., Valoski, A. M., Kalarchian, M. A., & McCurley, J. (1995). Do children lose and maintain weight easier than adults: A comparison of child and parent weight changes from six months to ten years. *Obesity Research, 3*, 411–417.

Epstein, L. H., Valoski, A. M., Vara, L. S., McCurley, J., Wisniewski, L., Kalarchian, M. A., et al. (1995). Effects of decreasing sedentary behavior and increasing activity on weight change in obese children. *Health Psychology, 14*(2), 109–115.

Epstein, L. H., Valoski, A., Wing, R. R., & McCurley, J. (1990). Ten-year follow-up of behavioral family-based treatment for obese children. *JAMA, 264*, 2519–2523.

Epstein, L. H., Valoski, A., Wing, R. R., & McCurley, J. (1994). Ten-year outcomes of behavioral family-based treatment for childhood obesity. *Health Psychology, 13*(5), 373–383.

Epstein, L. H., Wing, R. R., Koeske, R., Andrasik, F., & Ossip, D. J. (1981). Child and parent weight loss in family-based behavior modification programs. *Journal of Consultation and Clinical Psychology, 49*, 674–685.

Epstein, L. H., Wing, R. R., Koeske, R., Ossip, D. J., & Beck, S. (1982). A comparison of lifestyle change and programmed aerobic exercise on weight and fitness changes in obese children. *Behavior Therapy, 13*, 651–665.

Epstein, L. H., Wing, R. R., Steranchak, L., Dickson, B., & Michelson, J. (1980). Comparison of family based behavior modification and nutrition education for childhood obesity. *Journal of Pediatric Psychology, 5*, 25–36.

Epstein, L. H., Wisniewski, L., & Weng, R. (1994). Child and parent psychological problems influence child weight control. *Obesity Research, 2*, 509–515.

Erermis, S., Cetin, N., Tamar, M., Bukusoglu, N., Akdeniz, F., & Goksen, D. (2004). Is obesity a risk factor for psychopathology among adolescents? *Pediatrics International, 46*(3), 296–302.

Flegal, K. M., Carroll, M. D., Ogden, C. L., & Johnson, C. L. (2002). Prevalence and trends in obesity among U.S. adults. *JAMA, 288*, 1723–1727.

Goetz, D. R., & Caron, W. (1999). A biopsychosocial model for youth obesity: Consideration of an ecosystemic collaboration. *International Journal of Obesity, 23*(S2), S58–S64.

Golan, M., Weizman, A., Apter, A., & Fainaru, M. (1998). Parents as exclusive agents of change in the treatment of childhood obesity. *American Journal of Clinical Nutrition, 67*, 1130–1135.

Gortmaker, S. L., Cheung, L. W. Y., Peterson, K. E., Chomitz, G., Cradle, J. H., Dart, H., et al. (1999). Impact of a school-based interdisciplinary intervention on diet and activity among urban primary school children: Eat well and keep moving. *Archives of Pediatrics and Adolescent Medicine, 123*(9), 975–983.

Gortmaker, S., Must, A., Sobol, A., Peterson, K., Colditz, G., & Dietz, W. (1996). Television viewing as a cause of increasing obesity among children in the United States 1986–1990. *Journal of the American Medical Association, 150*(4), 356–362.

Jeffery, R. W., & French, S. A. (1998). Epidemic obesity in the US: Are fast foods and television viewing contributing? *American Journal of Public Health, 88*, 277–280.

Kelder, R. W., Perry, C. L., Klepp, K. I., & Lytle L. L. (1994). Longitudinal tracking of adolescent smoking, physical activity, and food choice behaviors. *American Journal of Public Health, 84*, 1121–1126.

Knip, M., & Nuutinen, O. (1993). Long-term effects of weight reduction on serum lipids and plasma insulin in obese children. *American Journal of Clinical Nutrition, 54*, 490–493.

Kohl, H. W., & Hobbs, K. E. (1998). Development of physical activity behaviors among children and adolescents. *Pediatrics, 101*, 549–554.

Kotz, K., & Story, M. (1994). Food advertisements during children's Saturday morning television programming: Are they consistent with dietary recommendations? *Journal of American Dietetic Association, 94*, 1296–1300.

Kraak, V., & Pelletier, D. L. (1998). The influence of commercialism on the food purchasing behavior of children and teenage youth. *Family Economy Nutrition Review, 11*, 15–24.

Lytle, L. A., Kelder, S. H., Perry, C. L., & Klepp, K. I. (1995). Covariance of adolescent health behaviors—The class of 1989 study. *Health Education Research Theory and Practice, 10*, 133–146.

Marshall, S. J., Biddle, S. J. H., Gorely, T., Cameron, N., & Murdey, I. (2004). Relationship between media use and body fatness and physical activity in children and youth: A meta-analysis. *International Journal of Obesity, 28*(10), 1238–1246.

National Center for Health Statistics. (1999). *Prevalence of overweight among children and adolescents: United States, 1999.* Retrieved July 2004, from http://www.cdc.gov/nchs/products/pubs/pubd/hestats/overwght99.htm

National Institute on Media and the Family. (2004). *Fact sheet: Media use and obesity among children.* Retrieved July 14, 2004, from http://www.mediafamily.org/facts/facts_tvandobchild_print.shtml

Ogden, C. L., Flegal, K. M., Carroll, M. D., & Johnson, C. L. (2002). Prevalence and trends in overweight among US children and adolescents, 1999–2000. *JAMA, 288*, 1728–1732.

Raue, P. J., Castonguay, L. G., & Goldfried, M. R. (1993). The working alliance: A comparison of two therapies. *Psychotherapy Research, 3*, 197–207.

Rees, J. M. (1990). Management of obesity in adolescence. *Medical Clinics of North America, 74*, 1275–1292.

Rimm, S. (2004). *Rescuing the emotional lives of overweight children: What our kids go through—and how we can help.* Emmaus, PA: Rodale.

Senediak, C., & Spence, S. H. (1985). Rapid versus gradual scheduling of therapeutic contact in a family based behavioural weight control programme for children. *Behavioral Psychotherapy, 13*, 265–287.

Serdula, M. K., Ivery, D., Coates, R. J., Freedman, D. S., Williamson, D. F., & Byers, T. (1993). Do obese children become obese adults? A review of the literature. *Preventive Medicine, 22*, 167–177.

TV Turnoff Network. (2004). TV turnoff week. Retrieved June 14, 2004, from http://www.tvturnoff.org/index.htm

Wadden, T. A., Foster, G. D., Brownell, K. D., & Finley, E. (1984). Self-concept in obese and normal-weight children. *Journal of Consulting and Clinical Psychology, 52*, 1104–1105.

Chapter 10

Botvin, G. J., Mihalic, S. F., & Grotpeter, J. K. (1998). *Life skills training.* Boulder, CO: Center for the Study and Prevention of Violence, Institute of Behavioral Science, University of Colorado.

Bracken, B. A. (1993). *Assessment of interpersonal relations.* Austin, TX: Pro-Ed.

Caldarella, P., & Merrell, K. W. (1997). Common dimensions of social skills of children and adolescents: A taxonomy of positive behaviors. *School Psychology Review, 26,* 264–278.

Caplan, M. Z., & Weissberg, R. P. (1988). Promoting social competence in early adolescence: Developmental considerations. In G. H. Schneider, G. Attili, J. Nadel, & R. P. Weissberg (Eds.), *Social competence in developmental perspective* (pp. 371–386). Boston: Kluwer Academic.

Cartledge, G. (1996). *Cultural diversity and social skills instruction: Understanding ethnic and gender differences.* Champaign, IL: Research Press.

Centers for Disease Control and Prevention. (2004, May 21). Surveillance summaries. *MMWR, 53* (No. SS-2).

DeRosier, M. E. (2004). Building relationships and combating bullying: Effectiveness of a school-based social skills group intervention. *Journal of Clinical and Adolescent Psychology, 33,* 196–201.

Dupper, D. R. (1998). An alternative to suspension for middle school youths with behavior problems: Findings from a "school survival" group. *Research on Social Work Practice, 8,* 354–366.

Dupper, D. R. (2003). *School social work: Skills and interventions for effective practice.* Hoboken, NJ: Wiley.

Dupper, D. R., & Krishef, C. H. (1993). School-based social-cognitive skills training for middle school students with school behavior problems. *Children and Youth Services Review, 15,* 131–142.

Elliott, S. N., & Gresham, F. M. (1991). *Social skills intervention guide: Practical strategies for social skills training.* Circle Pines, MN: American Guidance.

Greenberg, M. T., Kusche, C., & Mihalic, S. F. (1998). *Promoting alternative thinking strategies (PATHS).* Boulder, CO: Center for the Study and Prevention of Violence, Institute of Behavioral Science, University of Colorado.

Gresham, F. M. (1986). Conceptual issues in the assessment of social competence in children. In P. S. Strain, M. J. Guralnick, & H. M. Walker (Eds.), *Children's social behavior: Development, assessment, and modification* (pp. 143–179). New York: Academic.

Gresham, F. M. (2002). Best practices in social skills training. In A. Thomas & J. Grimes (Eds.), *Best practices in school psychology* (4th ed., Vol. 2, pp. 1029–1040). Bethesda, MD: National Association of School Psychologists.

Gresham, F. M., & Elliott, S. N. (1990). *The social skills rating system.* Circle Pines, MN: American Guidance.

Gresham, F. M., & MacMillan, D. L. (1997). Social competence and affective characteristics of students with mild disabilities. *Review of Educational Research, 67,* 377–415.

Gresham, F. M., Sugai, G., & Horner, R. H. (2001). Interpreting outcomes of social skills training for students with high-incidence disabilities. *Exceptional Children, 67,* 331–344.

Hoagwood, K., & Erwin, H. D. (1997). Effectiveness of school-based mental health services for children: A 10-year research review. *Journal of Child and Family Studies, 6*, 435–451.

Katz, L. G., McClellan, D. E., Fuller, J. O., & Walz, G. R. (1995). *Building social competence in children: A practical handbook for counselors, psychologist, and teachers.* ERIC Elementary and Early Childhood Education Clearinghouse. Washington, DC: U.S. Department of Education.

Krieg, F. J., Simpson, C., Stanley, R. E., & Snider, D. A. (2002). Best practices in making school groups work. In A. Thomas & J. Grimes (Eds.), *Best practices in school psychology* (4th ed., Vol. 2, pp. 1195–1216). Bethesda, MD: National Association of School Psychologists.

LeCroy, C. W. (Ed.). (1983). *Social skills training for children and youth.* New York: Haworth.

LeCroy, C. W. (1992). *Case studies in social work practice.* Belmont, CA: Wadsworth.

LeCroy, C. W. (2002). Child therapy and social skills. In A. R. Roberts & G. J. Greene (Eds.), *Social workers' desk reference* (pp. 406–412). New York: Oxford University Press.

LeCroy, C. W., & Wooten, L. E. (2002). Social skills groups in schools. In R. Constable, S. McDonald, & J. P. Flynn (Eds.), *School social work: Practice, policy and research perspectives* (pp. 441–457). Chicago: Lyceum.

Lochman, J. E., Lampron, L. B., Gemmer, T. C., Harris, S. R., & Wyckoff, G. M. (1989). Teacher consultation and cognitive-behavioral intervention with aggressive boys. *Psychology in the Schools, 26,* 179–188.

Lochman, J. E., & Wells, K. C. (1996). A social-cognitive intervention with aggressive children: Prevention effects and contextual implementation issues. In. R. DeV. Peters & R. J. McMahon (Eds.), *Preventing childhood disorders, substance abuse and delinquency* (pp. 111–143). Thousand Oaks, CA: Sage.

Lope, M., & Edelbaum, J. (1999). *I'm popular! Do I need social skills training?* Available: http://www.personal.psu.edu/faculty/j/g/jgp4/teach/497/social skillstraining.htm

Merrell, K. W. (1994). *Preschool and kindergarten behavior scales.* Austin, TX: Pro-Ed.

Merrell, K. W., & Gimpel, G. A. (1998). *Social skills of children and adolescents: Conceptualization, assessment, treatment.* Mahwah, NJ: Erlbaum.

Poland, S., Pitcher, G., & Lazarus, P. M. (2002). Best practices in crisis prevention and management. In A. Thomas & J. Grimes (Eds.), *Best practices in school psychology* (4th ed., Vol. 2, pp. 1057–1079). Bethesda, MD: National Association of School Psychologists.

Reynolds, C. R., & Kamphaus, R. W. (1992). *The behavioral assessment system for children.* Circle Pines, MN: American Guidance Services.

Rose, S. R. (1998). *Group work with children and adolescents: Prevention and intervention in school and community systems.* Thousand Oaks, CA: Sage.

Scott, D. (n.d.). *Program outcomes for youth: Social competence.* Available: http://ag.arizona.edu/fcs/cyfernet/nowg/social_comp.html.

Stein, J. A., Newcomb, M. D., & Bentler, P. M. (1992). The effect of agency and communality on self-esteem: Gender differences in longitudinal data. *Sex Roles, 26,* 465–483.

Walker, H. M., & McConnell, S. R. (1995). *The Walker-McConnell scales of social competence and school adjustment.* San Diego, CA: Singular.

Weissberg, R. P., Barton, H. A., & Shriver, T. P. (1997). The social competence promotion program for young adolescents. In G. W. Albee & T. P. Gullotta (Eds.), *Primary prevention works* (pp. 268–290). Thousand Oaks, CA: Sage.

Weissberg, R. P., Kumpfer, K. L., & Seligman, M. E. P. (2003). Prevention that works for children and youth. *American Psychologist, 58*, 425–432.

Index

National Institute on Drug Abuse
(NIDA), 43, 51
National Registry of Effective Prevention
Programs (NREPP), 5
National Survey on Drug Use and Health
(SAMHSA), 3
Negotiation skills
and HIV prevention, 73–74

Obsessive-compulsive disorder (OCD)
co-occurring disorders of
self-mutilation behavior, 88
Off-label use by physicians, 98
Opioid antagonists, 98
Oppositional defiant disorder (ODD)
co-occurring disorders of
self-mutilation behavior, 92
Outward Bound, *8*

Peers
for substance abuse (elementary
students), *22*
Personal Experience Screening
Questionnaire (PESQ), *49*
Physical abuse
co-occurring disorders of, 92
Positive Action (PA), 20, 26, *30*, 37–40,
39, 42
goal and objectives, 37–38
outcomes, 40
structure and implementation, 38–40
target population, 38
Post-traumatic stress disorder
co-occurring disorders of
self-mutilation behavior, 88
Prevention Enhancement Protocols
System (PEPS), *9*
Problem-Oriented Screening Instruments
for Teenagers (POSIT), 44, *50,*
51–52, 61n1
Problem-solving training
for self-mutilation behavior, 97,
101–102
Project ACHIEVE, *31*
Project Counseling Leadership About
Smoking Pressure (CLASP), *9*
Project DARE (Drug Abuse Resistance
Education), 4
Psychotic disorders
co-occurring disorders of

self-mutilation behavior, 88
Public service announcements, 4

Reducing the Risk, *67*
Risk factors
for STD prevention, 80
for substance abuse (elementary
students), 21–24, *21–23*
for substance abuse (middle and high
school students), 43
Runaway youth, 64, 78
Rutgers Alcohol Problem Index
(RAPI), 44, *50,* 51, *52–56,* 61n2

Safer Choices, *68*
Safety Contracts, 99, *100*
Screening
for substance abuse (middle and high
school students), 43–61, *57, 60*
key points, 61
practice examples, 58–61
screening, assessment, and
diagnosis, 45
screening instruments, 44–56,
46–51, 53, 56, 59, 61nn1–2
tools, 56
Selective serotonin reuptake inhibitors
(SSRIs)
for self-mutilation behavior, 98
Self Center, *68*
Self-mutilation behavior (SMB), 87–107
background research on, 87–93
compulsive SMB, 88
contagion factor, 93
factors associated with, 91–93
functions of, 89–90
impulsive SMB, 88, 91
major SMB, 88
personal accounts of, 90–91
prevalence of, 88–89
stereotypic SMB, 88
confidentiality issue, 94
co-occurring disorders of, 87–88,
91–92
depression, 88
post-traumatic stress disorder, 88
substance abuse, 87, 92
suicidality, 87
identification and assessment of, 93–94
interventions, 94–98